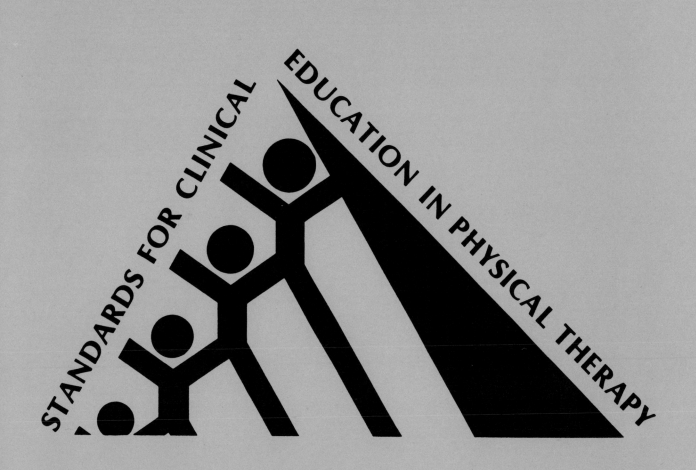

STANDARDS FOR CLINICAL EDUCATION IN PHYSICAL THERAPY

A MANUAL FOR EVALUATION AND SELECTION OF CLINICAL EDUCATION CENTERS

Jean S. Barr, Project Director
Jan Gwyer, Research Assistant
Zippora Talmor, Research Assistant

STANDARDS FOR CLINICAL EDUCATION
IN PHYSICAL THERAPY

A MANUAL FOR EVALUATION
AND SELECTION OF CLINICAL
EDUCATION CENTERS

by

Jean S. Barr, Project Director
Jan Gwyer, Research Assistant
Zippora Talmor, Research Assistant

Principal Investigators:

Margaret L. Moore, 1978-1979
Barry R. Howes, 1979-1980

Published by

American Physical Therapy
Association

1156 15th Street NW
Washington, DC 20005

1981

STANDARDS FOR CLINICAL EDUCATION
IN PHYSICAL THERAPY

Sponsored by:
        Department of Medical Allied Health Professions
        School of Medicine
        University of North Carolina at Chapel Hill
        Chapel Hill, North Carolina

Supported in part by:
        Department of Health, Education, and Welfare
        Public Health Service
        Health Resources Administration
        Bureau of Health Manpower
        Division of Associated Health Professions
        Allied Health Special Project
        Grant # 1 D12AH 90181

PREFACE

The purpose of this manual is to provide the physical therapy profession with a set of standards with evaluation forms for evaluating and selecting clinical education centers, as well as with data which support use of these particular standards and evaluation forms. The manual is divided into two major sections. The first section includes a copy of the standards along with a copy of three evaluation forms, as well as discussion of the use of the standards and each evaluation form. The second section contains a brief description of the testing procedures used to refine the standards and evaluation forms and presents the results of data collected about the standards and the reliability and validity of the evaluation forms and process.

In the Fall of 1978, the University of North Carolina at Chapel Hill was awarded a two-year Allied Health Special Project grant by the Department of Health, Education, and Welfare to study selection of clinical education centers in physical therapy. The purposes of the two-year project were to test, refine, and distribute standards and forms for evaluating centers for clinical education of physical therapist and physical therapist assistant students. Altogether, 857 physical therapists and 52 students participated in the research which led to the production of this manual. This project was initiated by the Section for Education of the American Physical Therapy Association and was based on work conducted earlier by the Section, under the leadership of Margaret L. Moore and Jan F. Perry, and reported in <u>Clinical Education in Physical Therapy: Present Status/Future Needs</u> (Moore and Perry, 1976).

The authors wish to acknowledge consultation about the overall design of the Project from Eugene Michels; consultation and assistance with data analysis from Richard T. Campbell; editing of the manual by Patrick A. Flannery; consultation about statistical tests and computer programming from Tom Novak, Donna Hoffman, and Kar Wang Lau; critiques of the manual by Suzann K. Campbell, Mabel M. Parker, Jan F. Perry, and Irma Wilhelm; and preparation of the manual by Linda Barton and Ellen Willard.

September 1980
Chapel Hill, North Carolina

Jean S. Barr
Jan Gwyer
Zippora Talmor
Margaret L. Moore
Barry R. Howes

GLOSSARY OF TERMS

Academic Coordinator of Clinical Education (ACCE)

An individual, employed by the educational institution, whose primary concern is relating the students' clinical education to the curriculum. This coordinator administers the total clinical education program and, in association with the academic and clinical faculty, plans and coordinates the individual student's program of clinical experience with academic preparation, and evaluates the student's progress.

Center Coordinator of Clinical Education (CCCE)

The individual at each clinical education center who coordinates and arranges the clinical education of the physical therapy student and who communicates with the ACCE and faculty at the educational institution. This person may or may not have other responsibilities at the clinical education center.

Clinical Education

The portion of the student's professional education which involves practice and application of classroom knowledge and skills to on-the-job responsibilities. This occurs at a variety of centers and includes experience in evaluation and patient care, administration, research, teaching, and supervision. It is a participatory experience with limited time spent in observation.

Clinical Education Center

A health care agency or other setting in which learning opportunities and guidance in clinical education for physical therapy students are provided. The clinical education center may be a hospital, agency, clinic, office, school, or home and is affiliated with one or more educational programs through a contractual agreement.

Clinical Instructor (CI)

A person who is responsible for the direct instruction and supervision of the physical therapy student in the clinical education setting.

Educational Institution

The academic setting in which the physical therapy educational program is located (e.g., university, college).

Educational Program

The academic entity responsible for the education of physical therapy students (e.g., school or department of physical therapy).

Level of Student

Beginning Level: first period of assignment in clinical education during basic professional preparation; often part-time assignments.

Advanced Level: intermediate or final period of assignment in clinical education during basic professional preparation; part-time or full-time assignments.

Graduate Level: a clinical experience during advanced professional preparation; related strictly to the graduate student.

Physical Therapy Service

The organizational entity responsible for the delivery of services (e.g., clinical department of a hospital).

Physical Therapy Student

Refers, when used in the general sense, to both physical therapist assistant and physical therapist students.

Definitions taken, in part, from the Final Report of the Project on Clinical Education in Physical Therapy, Moore and Perry, federal contract NO1-AH-44112, 1976.

TABLE OF CONTENTS

SECTION I: STANDARDS AND EVALUATION FORMS

I. A INTRODUCTION

A. 1 Standards as Characteristics

Data from the Project on Clinical Education indicated certain characteristics to be important as a basis for selection and retention of a clinical education center for the education of physical therapy students. These important characteristics have been organized into a list of 20 standards.

A. 2 Use of Standards

Extensive testing of the standards showed that the standards may be used equally well for the service with a small clinical staff and for the service with a large staff, as well as for the community-based or speciality program and the hospital-based program. The standards are guidelines to assist the ACCE in evaluating a clinical center prior to affiliating with an educational program and on a routine basis thereafter.

The standards are presented in two groups. Standards 1 - 5 were considered to be the most important by ACCEs and CCCEs. A satisfactory level of compliance with these standards should be achieved before accepting/assigning students in a clinical center. Standards 6-20 can be considered goals to work toward in achieving the most effective clinical education program.

A. 3 Uses of Evaluation Forms

A. 3. a <u>Self-Assessment of a Physical Therapy Clinical Education Center</u>

This inventory should be used by the physical therapy staff at the clinical center to evaluate their resources for planning and conducting clinical education programs. The self-assessment should then be reviewed by the ACCE at the educational program with which the center is or will be affiliated.

A. 3. b <u>Profile of a Physical Therapy Clinical Education Center</u>

After completing the self-assessment inventory, the physical therapy staff at the clinical center should review their findings and complete the profile evaluation form. Using this graph, the physical therapy staff can determine the extent to which

their center is in compliance with each of the
standards for a clinical education center. The
strengths and weaknesses of the clinical education
program should be summarized, as well as any changes the staff plans to make. The profile evaluation form may also be completed by the ACCE, following a center visit, or after reviewing a completed
student's evaluation form or a completed self-
assessment form.

A. 3. c <u>Student's Evaluation of a Clinical Education
Experience</u>

This evaluation of a clinical education experience should be used by students following each
clinical experience. The results of the evaluation
should be shared with the CIs at the center as well
as the ACCE at the educational program.

I. B STANDARDS FOR A CLINICAL EDUCATION CENTER IN PHYSICAL THERAPY

STANDARD 1: THE PHYSICAL THERAPY SERVICE PROVIDES AN ACTIVE, STIMU-
LATING ENVIRONMENT APPROPRIATE FOR THE LEARNING NEEDS OF THE STUDENT.

The desirable learning environment in the clinical center demonstrates characteristics of good management, high staff morale, harmonious working relationships, and sound interdisciplinary patient
management procedures. Less tangible characteristics are personnel
receptiveness, a variety of expertise, interest in newer techniques,
and involvement with other professionals outside of physical therapy.
The learning environment need not be elaborate, but should be dynamic
and challenging.

STANDARD 2: CLINICAL EDUCATION PROGRAMS FOR STUDENTS ARE PLANNED TO
MEET SPECIFIC OBJECTIVES OF THE EDUCATIONAL PROGRAM, THE PHYSICAL
THERAPY SERVICE, AND THE INDIVIDUAL STUDENT.

Planning for students should take place in meetings among the Center
Coordinator of Clinical Education (CCCE), the Clinical Instructors
(CIs), and the Academic Coordinator of Clinical Education (ACCE).
The clinical education objectives of the educational program and the
physical therapy service should be used in planning student learning
experiences. Students should participate in planning their learning
experiences according to mutually agreed-upon objectives. The staff
in the clinical center should be prepared to modify particular learning experiences to meet individual student needs, objectives, and
interests. A thorough orientation to the clinical education program
and the personnel of the clinical center should be planned for the
student. Evaluation of student performance is an integral part of
the learning plan. Opportunities for discussion of and feedback
about strengths and weaknesses should be scheduled on an ongoing
basis.

STANDARD 3: THE CLINICAL CENTER HAS A VARIETY OF LEARNING EXPERI-
ENCES AVAILABLE TO STUDENTS.

Students in clinical education are primarily concerned with delivery
of services to patients; therefore, the physical therapy service
must have an adequate variety and number of patients, and adequate
equipment resources available for the planned learning experience.
Although the primary commitment of students is to patient care,
learning experiences should cover administration, supervision, teaching, and research. Other learning experiences for students might
evolve from: rounds, case conferences, department meetings, team
meetings, planning sessions, special clinics, special educational
programs, observing in surgery, observing physicians in clinical
situations, participating in outpatient departments, bedside care,
clinic care, home care, and community activities. The range of
experiences with patients should include, when appropriate, screening,
evaluating, planning, treating, follow-up, and reporting.

3

STANDARD 4: THE PHYSICAL THERAPY STAFF PRACTICES ETHICALLY AND
LEGALLY.

All physical therapists and physical therapist assistants on the staff
should be practicing ethically and legally as outlined by the APTA
code of ethics, the state standards of practice, the state practice
act, and center policy. The center policy should include statements
on patients' rights, release of confidential information, photographic
permission, clinical research, and procedures for reporting unethical,
illegal, or incompetent practice of physical therapy to appropriate
authorities. All standards of practice should be in writing and
available to the staff and the students.

STANDARD 5: THE CLINICAL CENTER IS COMMITTED TO THE PRINCIPLE OF
EQUAL OPPORTUNITY AND AFFIRMATIVE ACTION AS REQUIRED BY FEDERAL LEG-
ISLATION.

The center must adhere to affirmative action policies and not knowingly discriminate on the basis of sex, race, color, religion, handicap, or national origin in recruiting, hiring, promoting, retaining,
training, or recommending benefits for or retirement of professional
or nonprofessional personnel. In addition, the center must not discriminate against students and must insure that each student is provided equal opportunities, learning experiences, and benefits.

STANDARD 6: THE CLINICAL CENTER'S PHILOSOPHY AND ITS OBJECTIVES FOR
PATIENT CARE AND CLINICAL EDUCATION ARE COMPATIBLE WITH THOSE OF THE
EDUCATIONAL INSTITUTION.

The clinical center and the physical therapy service should have a
written statement of philosophy including comments relating to their
responsibilities for patient care, community service and resources,
and educational and research activities. Clinical education objectives should be written specifically for the center by the center
staff. The philosophy and objectives of the clinical center and the
educational institution must be compatible, but not necessarily identical or in complete accord.

STANDARD 7: THE CLINICAL CENTER DEMONSTRATES ADMINISTRATIVE INTEREST
IN AND SUPPORT OF PHYSICAL THERAPY CLINICAL EDUCATION.

Administrative support can be demonstrated by a clinical center in
the following ways: a statement of commitment to clinical education
included in its philosophy; center policies regarding work time spent
in clinical education activities and compensation of staff for attendance at professional and continuing education meetings pertaining to
clinical education; written communication from the administrator of
the center and physical therapy staff indicating that they are interested, willing, and committed to sponsoring a program of clinical
education.

STANDARD 8: COMMUNICATIONS WITHIN THE CLINICAL CENTER ARE EFFECTIVE AND POSITIVE.

Effective and positive communications within the center can be demonstrated by: tables of organization to indicate formal lines of communication; regular meetings of staff and of advisory committees; informal oral and nonverbal communications with administrators, physicians, referral agencies, and patients; monthly and yearly reports listing staff activities and plans. Communication with or by students might fit the established patterns, or special arrangements might need to made.

STANDARD 9: THE PHYSICAL THERAPY STAFF IS ADEQUATE IN NUMBER TO PROVIDE A GOOD EDUCATIONAL PROGRAM FOR STUDENTS.

Adequate clinical education can be planned for a student in a center with one physical therapist or more. The adequacy of numbers relates to the number of students accepted and the nature of the learning experience. Student-staff ratio can vary according to the nature of the center and the nature of the staff, the level of the student, the type of student, and the length of the student's assignment.

STANDARD 10: ONE PHYSICAL THERAPIST WITH SPECIFIC QUALIFICATIONS IS RESPONSIBLE FOR COORDINATING THE ASSIGNMENTS AND ACTIVITIES OF THE STUDENTS AT THE CLINICAL CENTER.

Planning and implementing the clinical education program in the clinical center can be a joint effort of all clinical faculty. Because the relationship between the ACCE and the CCCE must be close, one physical therapist should be the key person for coordinating the clinical education program within the center. The physical therapist appointed as the CCCE should be proficient as a clinician, experienced in clinical education, interested in students, possess good interpersonal relationship and organizational skills, and be knowledgeable of the center and its resources.

STANDARD 11: CLINICAL INSTRUCTORS ARE SELECTED BASED ON SPECIFIC CRITERIA.

Clinical instructors should be interested in and willing to work with students. Normally, at least a year of experience should be a prerequisite for a CI, but in special programs or in special areas of expertise less experience has proven to be satisfactory. The CI should be proficient as a clinician. Personal characteristics of the CI should also be considered, including: enthusiasm, interpersonal relations, sensitivity to students, and receptiveness to suggestions.

STANDARD 12: CLINICAL INSTRUCTORS APPLY THE BASIC PRINCIPLES OF EDU-
CATION -- TEACHING AND LEARNING -- TO CLINICAL EDUCATION.

Clinical instructors should possess the ability to plan, conduct, and
evaluate a clinical education program based on sound educational
principles. Necessary educational skills include the ability to:
develop written objectives for a variety of learning experiences,
organize activities to accomplish these objectives, effectively supervise students to facilitate learning, and participate in a multifaceted process for evaluation of the clinical education program. To enable
the *CI to learn and then apply basic principles of teaching and
learning, the ACCE and the physical therapy staff should collaborate
on arrangements for presenting materials on clinical teaching to the
CIs.

STANDARD 13: SPECIAL EXPERTISE OF THE VARIOUS CENTER STAFF MEMBERS IS
SHARED WITH STUDENTS.

Clinical center staff members in physical therapy and in other professional disciplines related to physical therapy possess special expertise which can broaden the horizon and competency of students. This
special knowledge and expertise can be shared with students through
rotating systems of assignment, team meetings, departmental case conferences, inservice education programs, lectures, demonstrations, and
by observing individuals perform special procedures.

STANDARD 14: THERE IS AN ACTIVE STAFF DEVELOPMENT PROGRAM FOR THE
CLINICAL CENTER.

The staff development program should be in writing in the administrative manual stating policies concerning on-the-job training, inservice
education programs, continuing education program activities, attendance at state or national professional meetings, and graduate study.
Inservice education programs should be scheduled on a regular basis
and be planned by members of the staff. Student participation in
staff development activities should be encouraged.

STANDARD 15: THE PHYSICAL THERAPY STAFF IS INTERESTED AND ACTIVE IN
PROFESSIONAL ASSOCIATIONS RELATED TO PHYSICAL THERAPY.

Activities may include: self-improvement activities, professional
enhancement activities, professional activities relating to offices or
committees, papers or speeches presented, and other special activities.
It should be the policy of the center that the staff be encouraged to
be active professionally at local, state, and national levels. The
CI should provide students with information about professional meetings and encourage their participation.

STANDARD 16: THE PHYSICAL THERAPY SERVICE HAS AN ACTIVE AND VIABLE
PROCESS OF INTERNAL EVALUATION OF ITS OWN AFFAIRS AND IS RECEPTIVE
TO PROCEDURES OF REVIEW AND AUDIT APPROVED BY APPROPRIATE EXTERNAL
AGENCIES.

Evaluation of personnel should be completed at regularly scheduled
intervals and should include appropriate feedback to individuals.
Evaluation of the service by utilization review, peer review, or
medical audit should be required at regularly scheduled intervals.
Evaluations should be continuous and include all aspects of the service including research and teaching. The clinical education program
for various types and levels of students should be reviewed and
revised as changes in objectives, programs, and staff occur.

STANDARD 17: THE VARIOUS CONSUMERS ARE SATISFIED THAT THEIR NEEDS
FOR PHYSICAL THERAPY SERVICE HAVE BEEN MET.

Consumers of physical therapy services include patients and their
families, administrators, physicians and professional personnel,
referring agencies, and students. The degree of satisfaction from
all of these sources should be documented. For example, physicians
can express their satisfaction through increased or decreased referrals and increased or decreased reliance on the staff's judgment; and
student satisfaction can be assessed through the evaluation of their
clinical experience at the center.

STANDARD 18: ROLES OF THE VARIOUS TYPES OF PHYSICAL THERAPY PERSON-
NEL AT THE CLINICAL CENTER ARE CLEARLY DEFINED AND DISTINGUISHED
FROM ONE ANOTHER.

Current job descriptions reflecting the actual job being performed by
each individual and the role of the student while at the center
should be accessible to staff and students. Job descriptions should
reflect specific clinical education responsibilities of the staff.
Organizational charts should show the relationship of staff members
and to whom the student is responsible while at the center.

STANDARD 19: SELECTED SUPPORT SERVICES ARE AVAILABLE TO STUDENTS.

Support services which may be available should be documented in writing for the student prior to arrival and supplemented by additional
information upon arrival. Such support services might include:
health care, emergency medical care, and pharmaceutical supplies;
library facilities, educational media and equipment, duplicating service, and computer services; support from counseling personnel and
advisors in research design and independent study planning; room and
board, laundry, parking, special transportation, and recreational
facilities.

STANDARD 20: ADEQUATE SPACE FOR STUDY, CONFERENCES, AND TREATING PATIENTS IS AVAILABLE TO STUDENTS.

Those items of particular concern to students are: lockers for clothing and security of personal belongings, a study area, a charting area, adequate space for patient care activities, and a private area for counseling with a CI or other staff members. Classrooms and conference space may be available. They should be accessible for staff meetings, lectures, case conferences, and demonstration of activities.

SELF-ASSESSMENT OF A
PHYSICAL THERAPY
CLINICAL EDUCATION CENTER

PURPOSE

This inventory for self-assessment is designed to facilitate use of the
Standards for a Clinical Education Center in Physical Therapy. The assessment is intended to be useful to both the clinical center and the academic
institution for development of new clinical education centers and for
reassessment of existing clinical centers already utilized for physical
therapy students.

INSTRUCTIONS TO THE CENTER

1. Complete the items which are appropriate and applicable for your
    center. Throughout the inventory, please use "NA" to indicate those
    items which are not applicable or not appropriate to your center.

2. In completing this form, use the document, Standards for a Clinical
    Education Center in Physical Therapy, as guidelines.

3. When requested, please indicate if the written materials are available
    for review.

4. If the materials requested to be attached are not available, please
    explain.

5. Please attach additional pages when space is inadequate for your
    response.

IDENTIFICATION OF CENTER

A. 1. Name of center_____

A. 2. Address_____

_____

A. 3. Telephone_____

A. 4. Type of center_____

A. 5. Accreditation status including date and by whom_____

_____

A. 6. Name and address of Director of Physical Therapy*_____

_____

_____

A. 7. Center Coordinator of Clinical Education (Name)*_____

_____

COMPLETION OF SELF-ASSESSMENT

B. 1. Date Self-Assessment completed_____

B. 2. Signature of person responsible for completing Self-Assessment

_____

B. 3. Title_____

*Please attach copy of curriculum vitae

STANDARD 1

<u>THE PHYSICAL THERAPY SERVICE PROVIDES AN ACTIVE, STIMULATING ENVIRONMENT</u>
<u>APPROPRIATE FOR THE LEARNING NEEDS OF THE STUDENT.</u>

The desirable learning environment in the clinical center demonstrates characteristics of good management, high staff morale, harmonious working relationships, and sound interdisciplinary patient management procedures. Less tangible characteristics are personnel receptiveness, a variety of expertise, interest in newer techniques, and involvement with other professionals outside of physical therapy. The learning environment need not be elaborate, but should be dynamic and challenging.

1. a. Please evaluate the morale of the staff in the <u>physical therapy</u> <u>service</u>.

	Always high	Usually high	Sometimes high, sometimes low	Usually low	N.A.
1). Clerical staff	_____	_____	_____	_____	_____
2). Supportive personnel (i.e., aides, orderlies)	_____	_____	_____	_____	_____
3). Physical therapist assistants	_____	_____	_____	_____	_____
4). Physical therapists	_____	_____	_____	_____	_____

1. b. Please evaluate the morale of the staff in the <u>clinical center</u>.

	Always high	Usually high	Sometimes high, sometimes low	Usually low	N.A.
1). Administrators	_____	_____	_____	_____	_____
2). Nurses	_____	_____	_____	_____	_____
3). Occupational therapists	_____	_____	_____	_____	_____
4). Physicians	_____	_____	_____	_____	_____
5). Social workers	_____	_____	_____	_____	_____
6). Other_____	_____	_____	_____	_____	_____

	Yes	No
1. c. Do you have a manual for physical therapy administrative procedures?	____	____

	Yes	No

1. d. Would you characterize the physical
therapy staff as:

    1). being receptive to different ideas?   ____   ____
    2). possessing a variety of expertise?   ____   ____
    3). being interested in new treatment techniques?   ____   ____
    4). being involved with health professionals
        outside of physical therapy?   ____   ____

1. e. Do you consider staff turnover a problem:

    1). in your clinical center?   ____   ____
    2). in your physical therapy service?   ____   ____
    3). if yes, please explain below:

1. f. Please provide the information requested on the form on the
following page for each of the clinical instructors in your
service.

CLINICAL INSTRUCTORS PARTICIPATING IN CLINICAL EDUCATION
(PHYSICAL THERAPISTS AND PHYSICAL THERAPIST ASSISTANTS)

NAME	PT/PTA SCHOOL FROM WHICH GRADUATED	DEGREE(S) AND DATE(S) RECEIVED	YEARS OF:		CURRENT PRIMARY RESPONSIBILITIES (% OF TIME)					AREA(S) OF SPECIAL CLINICAL TRAINING/ EXPERIENCE/ PRACTICE; % OF TIME NOW SPENT IN AREA(S)	ELIGIBLE FOR APTA MEMBERSHIP (YES/NO)	LICENSED OR ELIGIBLE FOR LICENSURE (YES/NO)
			CLINICAL PRACTICE	CLINICAL TEACHING	PATIENT CARE	ADMINISTRATION	EDUCATION	RESEARCH	OTHER			

Adapted from the APTA Accreditation Handbook, 1979.

13

CLINICAL EDUCATION PROGRAMS FOR STUDENTS ARE PLANNED TO MEET SPECIFIC
OBJECTIVES OF THE EDUCATIONAL PROGRAM, THE PHYSICAL THERAPY SERVICE, AND
THE INDIVIDUAL STUDENT.

Planning for students should take place in meetings among the Center Coordinator of clinical Education (CCCE), the Clinical Instructors (CIs), and the
Academic Coordinator of Clinical Education (ACCE). The clinical education
objectives of the educational program and the physical therapy service should
be used in planning student learning experiences. Students should participate in planning their learning experiences according to mutually agreed-upon
objectives. The staff in the clinical center should be prepared to modify
particular learning experiences to meet individual student needs, objectives,
and interests. A thorough orientation to the clinical education program and
the personnel of the clinical center should be planned for the student.
Evaluation of student performance is an integral part of the learning plan.
Opportunities for discussion of and feedback about strengths and weaknesses
should be scheduled on an ongoing basis.

		Yes	No
2. a.	Does your physical therapy service have written objectives for clinical education?	____	____
	(If yes, please attach)		
2. b.	Have the director of the physical therapy service, the CCCE, and the CIs all been involved in the preparation of objectives for clinical education?	____	____
2. c.	Are the clinical education objectives flexible to accommodate:		
	1). the student's objectives?	____	____
	2). students at different levels?	____	____
	3). the educational program's objectives for specific experiences?	____	____
2. d.	Are all members of the physical therapy staff who will be involved with clinical education familiar with the educational program's objectives for the curriculum and for clinical education?	____	____
2. e.	Are the possible learning experiences for clinical education outlined in writing and available to the ACCE and to the student?	____	____

	Yes	No

2. f. Does the CCCE or the CI discuss with the student his/her objectives for this experience prior to finalizing the specific learning experiences?   ____ ____

2. g. Have the CCCE and the ACCE discussed the needs of the clinical center regarding the following items:

1). reference materials?   ____ ____
2). equipment?   ____ ____
3). educational media?   ____ ____
4). other?_____   ____ ____

_____

2. h. Are the arrangements as to schedule, length of time, arrival time, housing, transportation, and available learning experiences verified in writing prior to the arrival of the student?   ____ ____

2. i. Do you have organized procedures for orientation of students?   ____ ____

(over)

	Yes	No

2. j. During the student's orientation, are the following objectives, policies, and procedures made available to students:

    1). clinical center's objectives?   ____ ____
    2). physical therapy service objectives?   ____ ____
    3). administrative procedures?   ____ ____
    4). patient-care procedures or ethical standards of practice?   ____ ____
    5). procedure manual for clinical education?   ____ ____
    6). accident report?   ____ ____
    7). personnel policies?   ____ ____
    8). patient-care plans?   ____ ____
    9). monthly and annual reports?   ____ ____
    10). physical-therapy-service table of organization?   ____ ____
    11). other?_____   ____ ____

_____

2. k. 1). Are the CIs willing to provide feedback to students regarding evaluation of their performance?   ____ ____

    2). What methods are used to assure feedback to students?

2. 1. Are the CIs willing to complete a final form for evaluation of the student to be returned to the ACCE?   ____ ____

16

THE CLINICAL CENTER HAS A VARIETY OF LEARNING EXPERIENCES AVAILABLE TO STUDENTS.

Students in clinical education are primarily concerned with delivery of services to patients; therefore, the physical therapy service must have an adequate variety and number of patients, and adequate equipment resources available for the planned learning experience. Although the primary commitment of students is to patient care, learning experiences should cover administration, supervision, teaching, and research. Other learning experiences for students might evolve from: rounds, case conferences, department meetings, team meetings, committee meetings, planning sessions, special clinics, special educational programs, observing in surgery, observing physicians in clinical situations, participating in outpatient departments, bedside care, clinic care, home care, and community activities. The range of experiences with patients should include, when appropriate, screening, evaluating, planning, treating, follow-up, and reporting.

3. a. *Please evaluate the learning experiences available at your clinical center for each type and level of student.*

   Students: PT (physical therapist) PTA (physical therapist assistant)

   Level: B (beginning) first period of assignment in clinical education during basic professional preparation; often part-time assignments.

   A (advanced) intermediate or final period of assignment in clinical education during basic professional preparation; part-time or full-time assignments.

   G (graduate) a clinical experience during advanced professional preparation related strictly to a graduate student.

   In each box of the table please enter an E (excellent), A (adequate), or M (marginal) as an evaluation of the quality of the learning experience in your clinical center. If the learning experience is not available in your center, please leave that row blank.

   E (excellent) - patient and learning resources always provide excellent exposure for students

   A (adequate) - patient and learning resources usually provide adequate exposure for students

   M (marginal) - patient and learning resources occasionally provide acceptable exposure for students

(over)

(Standard 3 continued)

Learning Experiences	PT			PTA	
	B	A	G	B	A
Acute adult					
Acute children					
Chronic adult					
Chronic children					
Cardiac rehabilitation					
Respiratory rehabilitation					
Burn unit					
Amputees					
Mental retardation					
Other special programs					
Early intervention					
Screening patients					
Evaluating patients					
Planning treatment programs					
Implementing treatment programs					
Referral for out-of-hospital follow-up care					
Rounds					
Case conferences					
Team meetings					
Outpatient clinics					
Observation in surgery					

Learning Experiences	PT			PTA	
	B	A	G	B	A
Service given:					
-bedside					
-physical therapy service					
-home					
-outpatient clinic					
Department meetings					
Committee meetings					
Department planning sessions					
Special education programs					
Inservice education					
Teaching					
Developing teaching materials					
Supervision					
Administration					
Consultation					
Professional growth					
Independent study projects					
Inservice education (planning, presenting, or demonstrating)					
Continuing education (planning, presenting, demonstrating, budgeting)					
Program planning (determining need, manpower, budget, recruitment procedures)					

(over)

(Standard 3 continued)

Learning Experiences	PT			PTA	
	B	A	G	B	A
Communications skills (oral and written)					
Research activities:					
-Departmental					
-Student's own					
Interdepartmental relationships					
Interagency relationships					
Interpersonal relationships					
Interdisciplinary activities					
Community activities					
Others:					

(Standard 3 continued)

3. b. Please describe the equipment in the physical therapy department in relation to:

	Adequate	Inadequate	Comment
1). type of patients treated.	____	____	
2). physical therapy procedures.	____	____	
3). modern, up to date.	____	____	

	Yes	No
3. c. 1). Is the normal patient load of the physical therapy service adequate for the student affiliations?	____	____

2). If no, please explain.

THE PHYSICAL THERAPY STAFF PRACTICES ETHICALLY AND LEGALLY.

All physical therapists and physical therapist assistants on the staff should be practicing ethically and legally as outlined by the APTA code of ethics, the state standards of practice, the state practice act, and center policy. The center policy should include statements on patients' rights, release of confidential information, photographic permission, clinical research, and procedures for reporting unethical, illegal, or incompetent practice of physical therapy to appropriate authorities. All standards of practice should be in writing and available to the staff and the students.

	Yes	No
4. a. Do you have available at the physical therapy service:		
1). Code of Ethics and Guide for Professional Conduct of the American Physical Therapy Association?	___	___
2). State Practice Act?	___	___
4. b. 1). Does your physical therapy service have a written policy for ethical standards of practice?	___	___
2). Does the policy include:		
i). patient's Bill of Rights?	___	___
ii). release of confidential information?	___	___
iii). permission for photographing?	___	___
iv). clinical research (human rights)?	___	___
v). newspaper reporting?	___	___
4. c. Does the center have a mechanism for reporting:		
1). unethical practice?	___	___
2). illegal practice?	___	___
3). incompetent practice?	___	___

THE CLINICAL CENTER IS COMMITTED TO THE PRINCIPLE OF EQUAL OPPORTUNITY AND AFFIRMATIVE ACTION AS REQUIRED BY FEDERAL LEGISLATION.

The center must adhere to affirmative action policies and not knowingly discriminate on the basis of sex, race, color, religion, handicap, or national origin in recruiting, hiring, promoting, retaining, training, or recommending benefits for or retirement of professional or non-professional personnel. In addition, the center must not discriminate against students and must insure that each student is provided equal opportunities, learning experiences, and benefits.

	Yes	No
5. a. Does the center comply with federal legislation which in effect prohibits discrimination on the basis of race, color, religion, handicap, national origin, and sex?	____	____
5. b. 1). Will your center accept students regardless of sex, race, color, religion, handicap, and national origin?	____	____
2). Will each student be provided equal opportunities, learning experiences, and benefits?	____	____
3). Will each student's performance be evaluated without regard to sex, race, color, religion, handicap, and national origin?	____	____
4). In assignment of students to learning experiences where numbers must be limited, do you have a written non-discriminatory plan for assignment?	____	____

5. c. If your answer to any of the above questions was no, please explain your answer briefly below.

STANDARD 6

**THE CLINICAL CENTER'S PHILOSOPHY AND ITS OBJECTIVES FOR PATIENT CARE AND
CLINICAL EDUCATION ARE COMPATIBLE WITH THOSE OF THE EDUCATIONAL INSTITUTION.**

The clinical center and the physical therapy service should have a written
statement of philosophy including comments relating to their responsibilities
for patient care, community service and resources, and educational and
research activities. Clinical education objectives should be written specifically for the center by the center staff. The philosophy and objectives of
the clinical center and the educational institution must be compatible, but
not necessarily identical or in complete accord.

		Yes	No
6. a.	Is there a written statement of philosophy:		
	1). for the clinical center?	___	___
	2). for the physical therapy service?	___	___
6. b.	Are there written objectives:		
	1). for the clinical center?	___	___
	2). for the physical therapy service?	___	___
6. c.	Are there written long-range plans:		
	1). for the clinical center?	___	___
	2). for the physical therapy service?	___	___
6. d.	1). Do you have written procedures for patient-care plans?	___	___
	2). If yes, do the written procedures include a policy for:		
	i). referrals?	___	___
	ii). role of staff members?	___	___
	iii). role of students?	___	___

After reviewing the educational institution's philosophy, curriculum objectives, objectives for clinical education, and objectives for specific experiences:

6. e. Do you believe your center's philosophy and objectives are compatible
with those of the educational institution?

Yes____   No____   Partially____

6. f. Do you believe the physical therapy service philosophy and objectives
are compatible with those of the educational institution?

Yes____   No____   Partially____

<u>THE CLINICAL CENTER DEMONSTRATES ADMINISTRATIVE INTEREST IN AND SUPPORT OF</u>
<u>PHYSICAL THERAPY CLINICAL EDUCATION:</u>

Administrative support can be demonstrated by a clinical center in the following ways: a statement of commitment to clinical education included in
its philosophy; center policies regarding work time spent in clinical education activities and compensation of staff for attendance at professional
and continuing education meetings pertaining to clinical education; written
communication from the administrator of the center and physical therapy
staff indicating that they are interested, willing, and committed to sponsoring a program of clinical education.

	Yes	No
7. a. 1). Does your center or physical therapy service present inservice education pertinent to clinical education for physical therapy staff?	___	___

2). If yes, please list the inservice education programs pertaining to clinical education presented during the past one to two years.

7. b. Does your center provide support for physical therapy staff to attend programs of continuing education pertinent to clinical education, such as:

	Yes	No
1). financial support (e.g., per diem, travel)?	___	___
2). release time?	___	___

7. c. Does the administrative support given to the center coordinator of clinical education include appropriate:

	Yes	No
1). time?	___	___
2). special training?	___	___
3). financial support?	___	___
4). relief from patient care?	___	___
5). other?_____	___	___

(over)

(Standard 7 continued)

                                                              Yes   No

7. d. 1). Does your physical therapy service
           currently affiliate with other
           educational programs?   ____   ____

       2). If yes, with how many educational programs
           does your physical therapy service affiliate?

            i). physical therapist educational programs_____
           ii). physical therapist assistant educational programs_____

                                                              Yes   No

7. e. Are your physical therapy service and your
       center administration willing to enter into
       a written agreement with an educational
       program?   ____   ____

7. f. Are you satisfied with the degree of interest
       your center administrator has demonstrated
       in clinical education for physical therapy?   ____   ____

STANDARD 8

COMMUNICATIONS WITHIN THE CLINICAL CENTER ARE EFFECTIVE AND POSITIVE.

Effective and positive communications within the center can be demonstrated by: tables of organization to indicate formal lines of communication; regular meetings of staff and of advisory committees; informal oral and nonverbal communications with administrators, physicians, referral agencies, and patients; monthly and yearly reports listing staff activities and plans. Communication with or by students might fit the established patterns, or special arrangements might need to be made.

                                                                        Yes   No

8. a. Do you have a written table of organization:

   1). for the clinical center? (If yes, please attach.)   ____   ____
   2). for the physical therapy service? (If yes, please
       attach.)   ____   ____

8. b. Please evaluate the effectiveness of the communication between the physical therapy service and other services, and within the physical therapy service as: Very Effective; Adequate, but room for improvement; or Ineffective. Also, please describe methods used to maintain effective lines of communication by checking the blocks appropriate to your facility.

	CHECK ONE				CHECK AS MANY AS APPROPRIATE									
	Effectiveness				Type			Frequency			Methods			
Communication between Physical Therapy Service and	Very effective	Adequate	Ineffective	N.A.	Face-to-face Communication	Telephone Communication	Written Communication	Daily Interaction	Weekly Interaction	Monthly Interaction	Rounds	Conferences	Inservices	OTHER (Please explain)
Administrators														
Physicians														
Patients														
Nursing Service														
Occupational Therapy														
Referral Agencies														
Social Service														
OTHERS:														

(over)

(Standard 8 continued)

Communication within the Physical Therapy Service between	Effectiveness				Type				Frequency				Methods			
	Very effective	Adequate	Ineffective	N.A.	Face-to-face Communication	Telephone Communication	Written Communication		Daily Interaction	Weekly Interaction	Monthly Interaction		Rounds	Conferences	Inservices	OTHER (Please explain)
Director of Physical Therapy and staff																
Among all staff																
Physical Therapy staff and students																

28

THE PHYSICAL THERAPY STAFF IS ADEQUATE IN NUMBER TO PROVIDE A GOOD EDUCA-
TIONAL PROGRAM FOR STUDENTS.

Adequate clinical education can be planned for a student in a center with
one physical therapist or more. The adequacy of numbers relates to the
number of students accepted and the nature of the learning experience. Student-staff ratio can vary according to the nature of the center and the
nature of the staff, the level of the student, the type of student, and the
length of the student's assignment.

	Yes	No

9. a. 1). *Does your staff have adequate time,
          in addition to service responsibilities,
          to assume responsibility for education
          of students?*   ____   ____

     2). *If no, please explain.*

9. b. *What is your usual staff to student ratio for each level of student?*

     B (beginning): *first period of assignment in clinical
                       education during basic professional pre-
                       paration; often part-time assignments.*
     A (advanced) : *intermediate or final period of assign-
                       ment in clinical education during basic
                       professional preparation; part-time or
                       full-time assignments.*

     *Please <u>check</u> the box that indicates your usual ratio of staff to
     students.*

RATIO STAFF TO STUDENTS	PT		PTA	
	B	A	B	A
1 to 1				
1 to 2				
1 to 3				
other_____ _____				

29

STANDARD 10

ONE PHYSICAL THERAPIST WITH SPECIFIC QUALIFICATIONS IS RESPONSIBLE FOR COOR-
DINATING THE ASSIGNMENTS AND ACTIVITIES OF THE STUDENTS AT THE CLINICAL
CENTER.

Planning and implementing the clinical education program in the clinical center can be a joint effort of all clinical faculty. Because the relationship
between the ACCE and the CCCE must be close, one physical therapist should be
the key person for coordinating the clinical education program within the
center. The physical therapist appointed as the CCCE should be proficient as
a clinician, experienced in clinical education, interested in students, possess good interpersonal relationship and organizational skills, and be knowledgeable of the center and its resources.

                                                        Yes   No

10. a.   1). Is responsibility for the coordination
             of clinical education assigned to one
             physical therapist?   _____   _____

         2). If no, please describe the method for
             assigning responsibility for this
             function.

10. b.   Please list the criteria your physical therapy service uses to select
         a physical therapist to coordinate clinical education activities.

30

CLINICAL INSTRUCTORS ARE SELECTED BASED ON SPECIFIC CRITERIA.

Clinical instructors should be interested in and willing to work with students. Normally, at least a year of experience should be a prerequisite for a CI, but in special programs or in special areas of expertise less experience has proven to be satisfactory. The CI should be proficient as a clinician. Personal characteristics of the CI should also be considered, including: enthusiasm, interpersonal relations, sensitivity to students, and receptiveness to suggestions.

                                                        Yes   No

11. a. Have all of the physical therapy staff
        members who are responsible for
        clinical education of students demon-
        strated a willingness to participate
        in the clinical education program?   ____   ____

11. b. List the criteria your physical therapy service considers to be
        minimum for selecting a clinician to teach and supervise students.
        If the qualifications vary for different levels of students or for
        specific learning experiences, please explain.

STANDARD 12

CLINICAL INSTRUCTORS APPLY THE BASIC PRINCIPLES OF EDUCATION--TEACHING AND
LEARNING--TO CLINICAL EDUCATION.

Clinical Instructors should possess the ability to plan, conduct, and evaluate a clinical education program based on sound educational principles.
Necessary educational skills include the ability to: develop written objectives for a variety of learning experiences, organize activities to accomplish these objectives, effectively supervise students to facilitate learning, and participate in a multifaceted process for evaluation of the clinical
education program. To enable the CI to learn and then apply basic principles
of teaching and learning, the ACCE and the physical therapy staff should collaborate on arrangements for presenting materials on clinical teaching to the
CIs.

12. a.   Please define the CI's role in:

     1). Establishing objectives with students:

     2). Planning learning activities:

     3). Supervising students:

     4). Evaluating students' performance:

     5). Counseling students:

                                                      Yes   No

12. b.   Do the CIs participate in evaluation of   ____   ____
         the entire clinical education program?

12. c.   1). Do your clinicians have specific   ____   ____
             preparation prior to assuming respon-
             sibility for teaching, supervision,
             and evaluation of students?

         2). If no, should the academic institution   ____   ____
             offer a program to prepare CIs?

32

	Yes	No

12. d. Are the following resources available to assist your CIs in becoming more proficient in applying basic principles of education to clinical teaching:

1). release time to study on the job? ____ ____

2). library reference materials in education? ____ ____

3). conference proceedings related to clinical teaching? ____ ____

4). self-instructional packages? ____ ____

5). _Handbook for Physical Therapy Teachers_? ____ ____

6). inservice education programs with own staff as instructors? ____ ____

7). inservice education programs with physical therapy instructors from educational institutions? ____ ____

8). workshops sponsored by educational institution? ____ ____

9). consultation services available from educational institutions? ____ ____

10). other?_____ ____ ____

SPECIAL EXPERTISE OF THE VARIOUS CENTER STAFF MEMBERS IS SHARED WITH STUDENTS.

Clinical center staff members in physical therapy and in other professional disciplines related to physical therapy possess special expertise which can broaden the horizon and competency of students. This special knowledge and expertise can be shared with students through rotating systems of assignment, team meetings, departmental case conferences, inservice education programs, lectures, demonstrations, and by observing individuals perform special procedures.

13. a. With knowledge of the areas of expertise of the physical therapy staff members mentioned in question 1. f, please indicate which methods are used to share this expertise with students in your physical therapy service.

For each method of sharing expertise, please check one column to indicate the frequency of use in your physical therapy service.

Methods of Sharing	Frequently used	Occasionally Used	Never Used
rotating assignments			
team meetings			
case conferences			
inservice programs			
lectures			
demonstrations			
observing individuals			
other_____			
_____			

13. b. At your center, which professional disciplines related to physical therapy share their expertise with physical therapy students?

Disciplines | Area of Expertise | Methods most frequently used to share expertise with students

THERE IS AN ACTIVE STAFF DEVELOPMENT PROGRAM FOR THE CLINICAL CENTER.

The staff development program should be in writing in the administrative manual stating policies concerning on-the-job training, inservice education programs, continuing education program activities, attendance at state or national professional meetings, and graduate study. Inservice education programs should be scheduled on a regular basis and be planned by members of the staff. Student participation in staff development activities should be encouraged.

	Yes	No

14. a.   Does your clinical center or physical therapy service have a written policy for staff development?   ____   ____

14. b.   Does your staff development program include policies regarding:

    1). inservice education within the physical therapy service planned by members of the physical therapy staff?   ____   ____

    2). continuing education programs (planned and presented by staff at your clinical center)?   ____   ____

    3). support for physical therapy staff to attend continuing education or professional meetings away from your center, such as:

        i). financial support (e.g., registration, per diem, travel)?   ____   ____
        ii). release time?   ____   ____

    4). support for physical therapy staff to enroll in graduate work for credit, such as:

        i). financial support (e.g., tuition)?   ____   ____
        ii). release time?   ____   ____

14. c.   1). Is student participation in your staff development program encouraged?   ____   ____

    2). If yes, please describe how student participation is encouraged.

STANDARD 15

THE PHYSICAL THERAPY STAFF IS INTERESTED AND ACTIVE IN PROFESSIONAL ASSOCI-
ATIONS RELATED TO PHYSICAL THERAPY.

Activities may include: self-improvement activities, professional enhancement activities, professional activities relating to offices or committees,
papers or speeches presented, and other special activities. It should be
the policy of the center that the staff be encouraged to be active professionally at local, state, and national levels. The CI should provide students with information about professional meetings and encourage their
participation.

	Yes	No
15. a. Is your physical therapy staff encouraged to participate in professional association activities?	___	___

15. b.   Please list the professional associations
(e.g., APTA) in which your staff is active.

15. c.   While students are affiliating with you,
are they aware of your staff's involve-
ment in professional association activities? ___   ___

15. d.   1). While students are affiliating with
you, are they encouraged to participate
in professional association activities? ___   ___

2). If yes, please describe how student
participation is encouraged.

STANDARD 16

THE PHYSICAL THERAPY SERVICE HAS AN ACTIVE AND VIABLE PROCESS OF INTERNAL
EVALUATION OF ITS OWN AFFAIRS AND IS RECEPTIVE TO PROCEDURES OF REVIEW AND
AUDIT APPROVED BY APPROPRIATE EXTERNAL AGENCIES.

Evaluation of personnel should be completed at regularly scheduled intervals
and should include appropriate feedback to individuals. Evaluation of the
service by utilization review, peer review, or medical audit should be
required at regularly scheduled intervals. Evaluations should be continuous and include all aspects of the service including research and teaching.
The clinical education program for various types and levels of students
should be reviewed and revised as changes in objectives, programs, and staff
occur.

		Yes	No
16. a.	Do you prepare reports for the physical therapy service:		
	1). on a monthly basis?	___	___
	2). on an annual basis?	___	___
16. b.	If you prepare reports for the physical therapy service, do they include:		
	1). patient statistics?	___	___
	2). source and type of referrals?	___	___
	3). physical therapy procedures administered?	___	___
	4). physical therapy procedures as related to utilization and need of space?	___	___
	5). status of equipment?	___	___
	6). personnel in relation to number of patient visits and treatment procedures?	___	___
	7). teaching activities?	___	___
	8). staff activities (e.g., research, special projects)?	___	___
	9). other? list:_____	___	___

_____

| | Yes | No | If Yes, How often? (e.g., annually, bi-annually, quarterly, monthly) |

16. c. Do you have procedures for internal review and evaluation of the following:

1). administrative procedures? _____ _____ _____

2). physical therapy personnel? _____ _____ _____

3). types of service rendered? _____ _____ _____

4). physical therapy department objectives? _____ _____ _____

5). physical therapy department budget? _____ _____ _____

6). inservice education programs? _____ _____ _____

7). clinical education programs? _____ _____ _____

16. d. What methods are utilized for external review and evaluation?

1). Utilization review: _____

2). Medical audit: _____

3). Peer review: _____

4). Other: _____

STANDARD 17

THE VARIOUS CONSUMERS ARE SATISFIED THAT THEIR NEEDS FOR PHYSICAL THERAPY SERVICE HAVE BEEN MET.

Consumers of physical therapy services include patients and their families, administrators, physicians and professional personnel, referring agencies, and students. The degree of satisfaction from all of these sources should be documented. For example, physicians can express their satisfaction through increased or decreased referrals and increased or decreased reliance on the staff's judgment; and student satisfaction can be assessed through the evaluation of their clinical experience at the center.

                                                              Yes   No

17. a. Do you have an organized plan whereby
        the following consumers participate in
        evaluation of your physical therapy
        services:

        1). patients?   ____   ____
        2). patients' families?   ____   ____
        3). administrators?   ____   ____
        4). physicians?   ____   ____
        5). professional personnel (not   ____   ____
            physical therapy personnel)?
        6). referral agencies?   ____   ____
        7). students?   ____   ____
        8). others?_____   ____   ____

        _____

17. b. For those consumers who do participate in evaluation of your physical
        therapy services, please describe their degree of satisfaction with
        the physical therapy service.

	Highly Satisfied	Moderately Satisfied	Dissatisfied (Please explain below)
1). patients	____	____	_____
2). patients' families	____	____	_____
3). administrators	____	____	_____
4). physicians	____	____	_____
5). professional personnel (not physical therapy personnel)	____	____	_____
6). referral agencies	____	____	_____
7). students	____	____	_____
8). others____	____	____	_____

        _____

40

STANDARD 18

ROLES OF THE VARIOUS TYPES OF PHYSICAL THERAPY PERSONNEL AT THE CLINICAL CENTER ARE CLEARLY DEFINED AND DISTINGUISHED FROM ONE ANOTHER.

Current job descriptions reflecting the actual job being performed by each individual and the role of the student while at the center should be accessible to staff and students. Job descriptions should reflect specific clinical education responsibilities of the staff. Organizational charts should show the relationship of staff members and to whom the student is responsible while at the center.

	Yes	No
18. a. 1). Do you have a job description for each type of personnel in physical therapy?	____	____

18. a. 2). If no, please list the types of personnel in physical therapy.

18. b. Do the job descriptions include the clinical education responsibilities of the:

	Yes	No
1). CCCE?	____	____
2). CIs?	____	____

PLEASE attach examples of 18. b. 1 and 2

18. c. Does the organizational chart for the physical therapy service clearly show:

	Yes	No
1). the relationship of staff members?	____	____
2). to whom students are responsible while at the center?	____	____

18. d. Are the roles of the various physical therapy personnel clearly defined for the student? ____ ____

STANDARD 19

SELECTED SUPPORT SERVICES ARE AVAILABLE TO STUDENTS.

Support service which may be available should be documented in writing for the student prior to arrival and supplemented by additional information upon arrival. Such support services might include: health care, emergency medical care, and pharmaceutical supplies; library facilities, educational media and equipment, duplicating service, and computer services; support from counseling personnel and advisors in research design and independent study planning; room and board, laundry, parking, special transportation, and recreational facilities.

	Yes	No

19. a. Is the student given advance written information as to:

1). availability, limitations, and cost of support services? ____ ____

2). how to secure assistance in obtaining the services desired? ____ ____

19. b. Please give information relating to these services as applicable. If not provided, please indicate if assistance will be given to the student in locating the service elsewhere (e.g., room and board).

Support Service	Provided by center		Not provided but available		Estimated cost to student	Assistance available	Comments on limitations
	Yes	No	Yes	No			
1). Emergency medical care							
2). Health services							
3). Pharmaceutical supplies							
4). Room							
5). Board							
6). Laundry							
7). Parking							
8). Special transportation							
9). Library facilities							

42

Support Service	Provided by center		Not provided but available		Estimated cost to student	Assistance available	Comments on limitations
	Yes	No	Yes	No			
10). Educational media and equipment							
11). Duplicating service							
12). Research resources; equipment; statistical consultation; computer services							
13). Stipend or reimbursement for expenses							
14). Other							

STANDARD 20

ADEQUATE SPACE FOR STUDY, CONFERENCES, AND TREATING PATIENTS IS AVAILABLE TO STUDENTS.

Those items of particular concern to students are: lockers for clothing and security of personal belongings, a study area, a charting area, adequate space for patient care activities, and a private area for counseling with a CI or other staff members. Classrooms and conference space may be available. They should be accessible for staff meetings, lectures, case conferences, and demonstration of activities.

	Yes	No
20. a. 1). Is the space available for the exclusive use of the physical therapy service adequate for student affiliations?	____	____
2). If no, please explain.		

20. b. For the following list of space arrangements, check yes for those which are adequate. Check no if inadequate and describe the method of contending with existing arrangements.

	Yes	No	Comment
1). Lockers or place assigned to students to secure personal belongings	____	____	
2). Space to accommodate students for treating patients	____	____	
3). A designated charting area for students in or near the treatment area	____	____	
4). A quiet study area available for students:			
i). during working hours	____	____	
ii). after working hours	____	____	

	Yes	No	Comment

5). A designated private area
for counseling with the
CI   ____ ____

6). Classroom or conference
room for small group
sessions and staff
meetings   ____ ____

7). Lounge area available
to students   ____ ____

CHECKLIST FOR ATTACHMENTS REQUESTED
(Please check as appropriate)

Attachment	Attached	Not available	Not applicable
Curriculum Vitae:			
A.6 Director of Physical Therapy			
A.7 Center Coordinator of Clinical Education			
2.a Written objectives for clinical education			
Table of Organization:			
8.a.1 For the Clinical Center			
8.a.2 For Physical Therapy			
Job Descriptions:			
18.b.1 Center Coordinator of Clinical Education			
18.b.2 Clinical Instructors			

CHECKLIST OF MATERIAL AVAILABLE AT THE CLINICAL CENTER FOR REVIEW
(Please check indicating who may have access to existing materials.)

Item	Does not exist	Available for review by			
		Physical Therapy Director	Physical Therapy Staff	ACCE	Students
CENTER					
4.c Mechanism for reporting unethical, illegal, incompetent practice					
5.b.4 Non-discriminatory plan for student assignment					
6.a.1 Statement of philosophy					
6.b.1 Written objectives					
6.c.1 Long-range plans					
PHYSICAL THERAPY SERVICE					
1.c Manual for administrative procedures					
4.a.2 State practice act					
4.b.1 Policy for ethical standards of practice					
6.a.2 Statement of philosophy					
6.b.2 Written objectives					
6.c.2 Long-range plans					
6.d Written procedures for patient-care plans					
14.a Staff development plan					
16.a Monthly or annual reports					
17.a Consumer satisfaction plan					

PROFILE OF A
PHYSICAL THERAPY
CLINICAL EDUCATION CENTER

PURPOSE

This profile evaluation is designed to summarize the results of the self-
assessment inventory. The profile will provide a graphic, as well as narra-
tive, representation of the strengths and weaknesses of the clinical education program, as measured by the Standards for a Clinical Education Center
in Physical Therapy.

The profile evaluation should be useful to the:

   --Center Coordinator of Clinical Education (CCCE), director of the phy-
     sical therapy service, and administrators of the clinical center as a
     periodic evaluation of their program of clinical education;

   --Academic Coordinator of Clinical Education (ACCE) and director of
     physical therapy educational program as an evaluation of clinical edu-
     cation centers available or utilized for clinical education; and

   --Students in their selection of a clinical education center to meet
     their objectives and interests for clinical experience.

INSTRUCTIONS

To the Clinical Center: After completing the Self-Assessment, you and your
colleagues at the clinical center should summarize your own findings as to
strengths and weaknesses. In addition, you may want to indicate changes you
wish to initiate and how these changes will be effected.

To the Educational Program: After reviewing the Self-Assessment completed
by the clinical center and other relevant materials, and perhaps making a
personal visit to the center, your Academic Coordinator of Clinical Education may use this form to summarize the findings and report strengths and
weaknesses, suggestions for improvement, and other matters concerning the
status of the clinical center as a site for clinical education in physical
therapy. The profile evaluation may then serve as a final report and recommendation to the center.

IDENTIFICATION OF CENTER

A. 1. Name of center_____

A. 2. Address_____

_____

A. 3. Telephone_____

A. 4. Type of center_____

A. 5. Name and address of Director of Physical Therapy_____

_____

_____

A. 6. Center Coordinator of Clinical Education (Name)_____

_____

COMPLETION OF PROFILE EVALUATION

B. 1. Date Profile Evaluation completed_____

B. 2. Signature of person responsible for completing Profile Evaluation

_____

B. 3. Title_____

INSTRUCTIONS: Please refer to the Standards for a Clinical Education Center in Physical Therapy and invididual items on the completed Self-Assessment of a Physical Therapy Clinical Education Center when using this form. Determine the compliance of this clinical education center with each standard by drawing a vertical line at the end of each row at the appropriate point on the scale. You may mark anywhere along the line that you wish, using the terms noncompliance, questionable compliance, and compliance as guides. Shading the area to the left of the line drawn for each standard will create a bar graph effect. This should create a visual description of the strengths and weaknesses of the clinical education program at this center. Please remember that ACCEs and CCCEs consider standards 1-5 to be the most important.

STANDARD	NON-COMPLIANCE	QUESTIONABLE COMPLIANCE	COMPLIANCE
1 Learning Environment			
2 Program Planning			
3 Learning Experiences			
4 Ethical Standards			
5 Affirmative Action			
6 Compatible Philosophy and Objectives			
7 Administrative Support			
8 Effective Communication			
9 Staff Number			
10 Clinical Education Coordinator			
11 Clinical Instructor Selection			
12 Principles of Teaching and Learning			
13 Sharing Special Expertise			
14 Staff Development			
15 Professional Associations			
16 Internal Evaluation			
17 Consumer Satisfaction			
18 Personnel Roles			
19 Support Services			
20 Adequate Space			

SUMMARY

A. Strengths as a Clinical Education Center

B. Weaknesses as a Clinical Education Center

C. Suggestions for Strengthening Program for Clinical Education

D. Recommendation as a Clinical Education Center in Physical Therapy
   (Specify type and level of student and limitations, if any.)

E. Recommendation for Next Action and/or Communication

I. E   STUDENT'S EVALUATION OF A
                            CLINICAL EDUCATION EXPERIENCE

PURPOSE

After each student's clinical experience with each center is completed, the
Academic Coordinator of Clinical Education and the Center Coordinator of
Clinical Education evaluate the affiliation and consider suggestions for
improvement. Students' opinions are an important part of this evaluation
process. Your positive, as well as negative, comments are very helpful.

INSTRUCTIONS

Please complete this evaluation at the end of your clinical education experience at this center. Place a check ($\checkmark$) in all appropriate spaces. Some
questions may not apply to your clinical education experience because of the
type of center or the length of time you spent at the center. In these
instances, please use the not applicable (NA) response. Please share the
completed evaluation with your Clinical Instructor(s) before returning the
evaluation to the Coordinator of Clinical Education at your *Educational
Institution*.

_____   _____

Name - Clinical Education Center   Dates of Clinical Education Experience

INFORMATION PROVIDED ABOUT THE CLINICAL CENTER

1. Please describe the following information or opportunities made available to you <u>prior</u> to your clinical education experience by the Coordinator of Clinical Education at your *Educational Institution*.

	Was not available; would not have been helpful	Was not available; would have been helpful	Was available; of little or no help	Was available; definitely helpful	N.A.
a. Facility & Administration					
1). Location	——	——	——	——	——
2). Visit to the center	——	——	——	——	——
3). Identification of staff	——	——	——	——	——
4). Met center staff	——	——	——	——	——
5). Personnel policies	——	——	——	——	——
6). Written agreements	——	——	——	——	——
b. Clinical Experience					
1). Type of patients served	——	——	——	——	——
2). Specialty programs	——	——	——	——	——
3). Objectives	——	——	——	——	——
4). Learning experiences	——	——	——	——	——
5). Length of affiliation time center requires	——	——	——	——	——
c. Information Pertaining to Students					
1). Support services available (i.e., Room, Board, Laundry)	——	——	——	——	——
2). Cost to student	——	——	——	——	——
3). Uniform requirements	——	——	——	——	——
4). Evaluation of center and recommendations from previous students	——	——	——	——	——

54

2. Please describe the following information made available to you prior to your clinical education experience by the Coordinator of Clinical Education *at your* *clinical center.*

	Was not available; would not have been helpful	Was not available; would have been helpful	Was available; of little or no help	Was available; definitely helpful	N.A.
a. Room and Board	___	___	___	___	___
b. Cars and Parking	___	___	___	___	___
c. Emergency medical care	___	___	___	___	___
d. Person to contact if any assistance is needed	___	___	___	___	___
e. Library facilities	___	___	___	___	___
f. List of staff	___	___	___	___	___
g. Location and time of first appointment	___	___	___	___	___
h. Optional learning experiences	___	___	___	___	___
i. Personnel policies	___	___	___	___	___
j. Rules & regulations	___	___	___	___	___
k. Schedule of working hours	___	___	___	___	___
l. Special meetings or programs	___	___	___	___	___
m. Directions to center	___	___	___	___	___
n. Uniform regulations	___	___	___	___	___
o. Other_____	___	___	___	___	___

_____

ORIENTATION

3. After your arrival at the center, were written objectives, policies, and procedures made available to you during your orientation:

	Yes	No
a. clinical center's objectives?	___	___
b. physical therapy service objectives?	___	___
c. administrative procedures?	___	___
d. patient-care procedures or ethical standards of practice?	___	___
e. procedure manual for clinical education?	___	___
f. accident report?	___	___
g. personnel policies?	___	___
h. patient-care plans?	___	___
i. monthly and annual reports?	___	___
j. physical therapy service table of organization?	___	___
k. other_____		

_____

4. Were you given adequate orientation to actual
   individual patients and responsibilities
   immediately prior to having the responsibility
   delegated to you?   Yes_____   No_____

5. After the orientation, did you, as well as your
   Clinical Instructors, have a clear understanding
   as to what was expected of you?   Yes_____   No_____

6. a. How would you describe the orientation you
      received?

         Adequate_____   Somewhat lacking_____   Totally inadequate_____

   b. If not adequate, please give suggestions for improvement.

LEARNING EXPERIENCES

7. Were the objectives for this center, as available
   to you preceding this affiliation, a true picture
   of the center and your actual experiences?   Yes_____   No_____

8. Were your objectives for clinical education
   considered in planning your learning experiences?   Yes_____   No_____

9. Did you feel that the learning experiences at this
   center were:

   a. Routine for every student who affiliated with
      this Physical Therapy service, or
   b. Modified for each student after considering
      the student's own previous experience and
      objectives?   a._____   b._____

10. Were on-going changes made in your learning
    experiences based on the level of competency
    you demonstrated?   Yes_____   No_____

56

11. Did you participate in preparing the following records or reports:

	Yes	No	N.A.
a. initial notes including evaluation notes?	____	____	____
b. progress notes?	____	____	____
c. development of patient-care plan?	____	____	____
d. discharge notes?	____	____	____
e. referral to other services?	____	____	____
f. referral to other centers?	____	____	____
g. home care programs?	____	____	____
h. problem oriented records?	____	____	____
i. internal audit or records?	____	____	____
j. external peer review?	____	____	____
k. attendance or ledger records?	____	____	____
l. other?_____			

_____

12. Did you have an opportunity to interact with members of other services for consultation, discussion, conferences, rounds, or lectures:

	Yes	No	N.A.
a. dietetics?	____	____	____
b. medical technology?	____	____	____
c. nursing service?	____	____	____
d. occupational therapy?	____	____	____
e. orthotics and prosthetics?	____	____	____
f. patient education?	____	____	____
g. medicine/surgery?	____	____	____
h. radiology?	____	____	____
i. social services?	____	____	____
j. speech therapy?	____	____	____
k. vocational counseling?	____	____	____
l. other?_____			

_____

13. While you were affiliating with this clinical
    education center, did you have an opportunity
    to meet:

    a. Students affiliating from other physical
       therapist or physical therapist assistant
       programs?   Yes_____ No_____
    b. Students who were affiliating with other
       departments within the clinical center?   Yes_____ No_____

    If yes, please identify by discipline:

                                                    Yes   No

14. Did you attend or present inservice
    education programs available to the physical
    therapy staff?

                                          Attended _____   _____

                                         Presented _____   _____

15. Were you provided with space adequate
    to accommodate your needs: Yes   No

    a. lockers or space to secure personal
       belongings?   _____   _____
    b. patient treatment area?   _____   _____

    c. charting and record keeping?   _____   _____
    d. quiet study area?   _____   _____

    e. private area for counseling with
       clinical instructors?   _____   _____
    f. small group conferences?   _____   _____
    g. lounge areas?   _____   _____

    h. other?_____
       _____

16. a. How would you describe your patient load during the majority of your
       clinical education experience?

       Appropriate for your level of education____ Too high____ Too low____

    b. Please comment if too high or too low:

17. a. Were the variety of patients adequate for you
       to meet the objectives of the clinical edu-
       cation experience?   Yes____ No____

    b. If no, please comment:

18. Was the equipment of the Physical Therapy
    Service adequate to meet the objectives of
    the clinical education experience?   Yes____ No____

    If no, please comment:

SUPERVISION

19. Did you have a clear understanding as
    whom you were directly responsible to?   Yes____ No____

20. a. Did you have adequate opportunity for
       communication with the clinical
       instructor to whom you were responsible?   Yes____ No____

    b. Please describe your opportunities for discus-
       sion with your clinical instructor by check-
       ing as many responses as are appropriate:

       Daily____; Once per week____; Whenever necessary____;

       Whenever requested____; Had to be scheduled in advance____;

       Impromptu____; Seldom____; Never____.

21. After the clinical instructor became familiar with
    your level of proficiency, were you given adequate
    opportunity to "try your wings"?   Yes____ No____

22. a. Based on your experience and skill, how would
       you describe the degree of supervision you
       received?

       Too close____ Commensurate with need____ Not close enough____

    b. If not commensurate with your need, please comment:

EVALUATION PROCESS

23. How frequently did you receive feedback on your clinical performance?

    Daily or whenever appropriate____ Midway____ Final____

24. How would you describe the final evaluation of your performance?

a. Discussed with you _prior_ to completion in writing so that you had an opportunity for discussion before it was finalized _____

b. Discussed before completion in writing, but with no opportunity to see the final form _____

c. Discussed after completion in writing _____

d. Not discussed _____

AFFIRMATIVE ACTION

25. Did this clinical center comply with the principles of equal opportunity and affirmative action as required by Federal legislation?

Yes_____ No_____ Do not know_____

If no, please cite examples of noncompliance:

PRIOR PREPARATION

26. What do you believe were the strengths and weaknesses of your academic preparation for this clinical experience?

Strengths:

Weaknesses:

27. Identify any new subject matter to which you were exposed during this clinical education experience and indicate if it should be included in the physical therapy educational program.

28. Based on your past experience in clinical education, and your concept of the "ideal" clinical education experience, how would you rate the clinical education experience at <u>this</u> clinical center?

1	2	3	4
A very negative experience; would not recommend to other students	A waste of time	Time well spent	A very positive experience; wish they all were like this

29. Please summarize your comments and make recommendations for this clinical education center.

Summary:

Recommendations:

_____   _____
            Student   Clinical Instructor/
                                                    Center Coordinator of
                                                    Clinical Education

Addendum comments by CCCE/CI:

SECTION II. STUDIES OF STANDARDS, EVALUATION FORMS, AND EVALUATION PROCESS

II. A INTRODUCTION

A purpose of the Project on Clinical Education was to provide the physical therapy profession with a set of standards that are clear, practical, reliable, and valid, and which can be used with all sizes and types of clinical centers, as well as stages and lengths of clinical education assignments. This purpose was achieved in a series of six separate studies. Together, the six studies involved a total of 134 Academic Coordinators of Clinical Education (ACCEs), 708 Center Coordinators of Clinical Education (CCCEs), 15 Clinical Instructors (CIs), and 52 students from across the country.

The first chapter of this section, Testing Procedures, will outline briefly each of the six studies giving information on the purpose, sample and response rate, and a review of the methods used. (For a more detailed discussion of methods see Barr, Gwyer, and Talmor, 1980a). The following three chapters will present results of studies of the standards, and reliability and validity of the evaluation forms and the evaluation process.

The results of our studies indicate that the 1980 Standards and Evaluation Forms should be used as described. If changed, adapted, or partial documents are used, they cannot be supported by the data reported here.

II. B TESTING PROCEDURES

Participants in the Pretest, Profile, and Weighting studies (described below) evaluated the "Standards for a Clinical Education Site in Physical Therapy" (1976 Standards) and accompanying evaluation forms reported in Clinical Education in Physical Therapy: Present Status/Future Needs (Moore and Perry, 1976). Revised (1980) Standards and Evaluation Forms, as they appear in this manual, were used by participants in the Interrater Reliability and Internal Consistency studies and test phase.

B. 1 Pretest

The purpose of the Pretest was to collect specific data regarding the clarity and practicality of the 1976 Standards and accompanying evaluation forms. Participants closely involved with physical therapy clinical education (i.e., ACCEs, CCCEs, and students) were asked to review the Standards or to use one or more of the forms to evaluate a clinical education center.

The Pretest design consisted of 14 cells: both physical therapist assistant (PTA) and physical therapist (PT) educational programs by seven different size/type categories of clinical education centers. Two sets of data per cell were desired. Thus, twenty-eight cells were planned. Each cell consisted of one ACCE and one student from a PT or PTA educational program, and one CCCE representing one of the seven center categories. A participant used and then critiqued the form(s) appropriate for him as outlined in Moore and Perry (1976). Critiques of the forms were collected through telephone interviews with each of the 84 participants.

B. 2 Profile Study

The purpose of the Profile study was to solicit from ACCEs and CCCEs individualized lists of characteristics that differentiate strong and weak clinical education centers and the rank order of the importance of the characteristics. It was assumed that these characteristics would provide information about implicit or explicit criteria currently being used by ACCEs or that CCCEs believe should be used by ACCEs to evaluate centers for clinical education of physical therapy students.

An open-ended Profile questionnaire was mailed to a random sample of 89 ACCEs of PT and PTA educational programs and 128 CCCEs. A 68 percent return rate was obtained. Thirty-eight characteristics of a "strong" (i.e., high quality) clinical education center were identified.

B. 3 Weighting Study

The primary purpose of the Weighting study was to assign a specific weight to each of the 1976 Standards or to arrange them in a particular order. A questionnaire was designed to assess whether some Standards were more important ("indicative of significant worth or value") and practical ("capable of being put to use") than others, which, if any, Standards were crucial ("important or essential..."), and whether to add or delete Standards.

The Weighting Critiques were mailed to three samples, consisting of 71 ACCEs and two random samples of 200 CCCEs each. Responses were obtained from 63 (88.7%) ACCEs and from 126 (63%) and 127 (63.5%) of each of the two CCCE samples.

In addition to the Weighting questionnaire, the two samples of CCCEs were used to answer two questions: 1) how important and practical the Standards are in the centers, and 2) Is there any communication between the ACCEs and CCCEs (i.e., do the CCCEs know how the ACCEs view the importance and practicality of the Standards)? One sample of CCCEs responded to the first question (responses designated "CCCE-center"); while the second sample answered the second question (responses designated "CCCE-academic"). Except for these response perspectives, all items included in the questionnaires of the two groups of CCCEs were identical.

B. 4 Interrater Reliability Study

The Interrater Reliability study was designed to study the reliability of the revised forms used to evaluate clinical education centers in physical therapy. Five centers which affiliate with a number of educational programs were chosen for the study. The CCCE, several CIs, and several students who had been assigned to that center, were asked to independently complete revised Self-Assessment, Profile, and Student's forms, respectively. Because of the difficult logistical problems in locating and getting cooperation from a large (n=10) and disparate group of professionals (CCCE, CIs, and students) all from one center, it was necessary to limit this study to a small number of centers. Although five centers were selected and agreed to participate, one dropped out during the data collection phase. In a second center, one of the CI questionnaires was lost in the mail, and one of the student questionnaires from a third center was not returned. Thus, three centers provided responses from one CCCE and four CIs and a fourth yielded data from the CCCE and three CIs. All five centers originally selected provided student data; four of them yielding responses from five students each, while a fifth provided data from four students.

This data set provided the opportunity to compare actual responses within a given center both within the clinical staff and between staff and students. The small n did not permit the calculation of the usual internal consistency measures, but the actual agreement across items was calculated as a measure of interrater reliability.

B. 5 Internal Consistency Study

While the Interrater Reliability study provided important information about the degree to which independent raters agree on evaluations within a given center, the small sample size did not permit the use of internal consistency approaches to the estimation of reliability. Moreover, the respondents in Interrater Reliability study were not independent, that is, each of the centers was rated by more than one rater. Although the CCCE and four CIs in each of the four centers being rated worked independently, the data from the 19 respondents refer to only four centers. Thus, the usual assumption of independence required in the calculation of internal consistency measures, such as Cronbach's Alpha, could not be met. To deal with this problem, 100 centers were selected at random and the CCCE in each center was asked to complete a revised Self-Assessment form. This sample and the analysis of data differed from the Interrater Reliability study by focusing on the perception of a center by only the CCCE, by potentially including all sizes and types of centers, and by comparing responses across centers. Exactly one-half of the sample responded.

B. 6 Test

The Test phase was planned to collect data that would demonstrate the reliability and validity of the clinical center evaluation process. It was hypothesized that the process, based on use of the 1980 Standards and Self-Assessment and Profile forms, was reliable (i.e., consistent across raters), and should be useful to ACCEs in evaluating clinical centers. It was further hypothesized that the process was valid (i.e., using this process will result in evaluations which are more discriminating and closer to an unbiased score, than evaluations based on personal perceptions of a center's reputation and varying amounts and kinds of information about the center).

The sample for this study consisted of 17 CCCEs (85% response rate), 43 ACCEs (80% response rate), and three project staff members. Each CCCE participant completed and returned a revised Self-Assessment form along with an estimate of the time required to complete it. Completed Self-Assessments were retyped, removing all identifying information and omitting any attachments which might identify the center. ACCE participants were asked to complete a series of two mail questionnaires. The function of the questionnaires was to have the ACCE rate a

clinical education center under two different conditions.
To guide their ratings, with the first questionnaire, the
ACCEs received a Self-Assessment form completed by a center
known to them. The identity of the center was withheld. With
the second questionnaire, the identity of the center and the
CCCE were given, but no Self-Assessment information was provided. Three project staff members also rated all 17 clinical
education centers after reading the Self-Assessment information provided by the center.

II. C STUDIES OF STANDARDS

To develop standards for clinical education which would be acceptable to the physical therapy profession, the following aspects of the 1976 Standards were studied: clarity, overlap, need, usefulness, order, and content validity. Data pertinent to each of these aspects is presented and discussed briefly in the following pages of this section. The 1976 Standards were revised based on these data resulting in the 1980 Standards which appear in Section I of this manual. (See Barr, Gwyer, and Talmor, 1980b for another presentation of results of Project studies.)

C. 1 Studies of 1976 Standards

C. 1. a Clarity and Overlap

The Pretest participants (28 CCCEs and 28 ACCEs) read and critiqued the 1976 Standards. The participants agreed that all 20 standards were clearly written and that the interpretation accompanying each standard, except standard 12--Principles of Teaching and Learning, helped to clarify the intent and scope of the standard. Six standards were found to have interpretations that overlapped; two of these, to have interpretations not pertinent to clinical education; and three additional interpretations did not pertain to clinical education. Editorial changes suggested by 10 percent or more of the Pretest participants were made in the 1976 Standards and interpretations.

C. 1. b Need

The need for standards by ACCEs and CCCEs was also investigated in the Pretest. The data show that standards are needed by ACCEs and CCCEs (Table 1).

Further analyses of the data were conducted to determine if standards would be appropriate in all settings used for physical therapy clinical education. The mean scores of the CCCEs by size and type of centers (Table 2) were compared. No significant difference among means was found using an F test at $p \leq .05$. These data indicated that standards for clinical education are needed by CCCEs regardless of the size of type of center. Sixty-nine percent of the ACCE and CCCE participants in the Pretest agreed that such standards should be used as guidelines rather than as minimal requirements (Table 3).

TABLE 1

NEED FOR STANDARDS REPORTED BY ACCES AND CCCES

| Respondent | Number | Mean Score[a] | |
		Standards needed by ACCEs	Standards needed by CCCEs
CCCEs	28	4.5	4.5
PT ACCEs	14	4.8	4.5
PTA ACCEs	14	4.6	4.4
TOTAL	56	4.6	4.5

[a]Scale: 1 = strongly disagree; 5 = strongly agree

TABLE 2

CCCE'S EXPRESSED NEED FOR STANDARDS BY SIZE/TYPE CATEGORIES

Size/Type of Centers	Number	Mean Score[a]
General Hospital > 400 beds	6	4.1
General Hospital < 400 beds	4	4.3
Rehabilitation Hospital	4	4.8
Other Hospital (Mental, Childrens)	3	4.7
Extended Care Facilities	4	4.5
Speciality Out-Patient with Clinic Setting (Private Practice, Daycare)	4	3.8
Community, Public, or Mental Health Without Clinic Setting	3	4.3

[a] *Scale: 1 = strongly disagree; 5 = strongly agree*

TABLE 3

USE OF STANDARDS AS GUIDELINES OR MINIMAL REQUIREMENTS

Participants	Number	Guidelines n (%)	Minimal Requirements n (%)
CCCEs	26	20 (77)	6 (23)
PT ACCEs	14	8 (57)	6 (43)
PTA ACCEs	14	9 (64)	5 (36)
TOTAL	54	37 (69)	17 (31)

C. 1. c Usefulness

The usefulness of the Standards was investigated in the Weighting study. ACCE and CCCE participants were given the list of 1976 Standards and asked whether they could be implemented in centers providing clinical education and to indicate the current frequency of use of the standards. Eighty-one percent of the ACCEs indicated that the Standards could be implemented in the centers they use for clinical education compared to a response of 87 percent from the CCCEs; 95 percent of the ACCEs reported using some or all of the Standards compared to 93 percent of the CCCEs.

Table 4 summarizes the frequency of use of each standard by ACCEs and CCCEs. Comparison of the ACCEs' and CCCEs' responses (recorded in the "Often/Very Often" column) shows that ACCEs believe that standards 5--Affirmative Action, 13--Sharing Special Expertise, 14--Staff Development, 15--Professional Associations, 16--Internal Evaluation, 17--Consumer Satisfaction, and 18--Personnel Roles are less often used in clinical education centers, while CCCEs report that these standards are used often.

TABLE 4

FREQUENCY OF USE OF EACH OF THE STANDARDS BY ACCES AND CCCES[a]

Standard Key Words	Not/Rarely Used		Used From Time to Time		Often/Very Often Used	
	ACCEs	CCCEs	ACCEs	CCCEs	ACCEs	CCCEs
	n[b] (%)	n (%)	n (%)	n (%)	n (%)	n (%)
Learning Environment	1 (2)	0 (0)	4 (7)	10 (4)	54 (91)	223 (96)
Program Planning	1 (2)	6 (2)	4 (7)	32 (14)	55 (91)	194 (84)
Learning Experiences	0 (0)	2 (1)	2 (3)	9 (4)	58 (97)	220 (95)
Ethical Standards	1 (2)	1 (0)	2 (3)	9 (4)	57 (95)	223 (96)
Affirmative Action	11 (18)	3 (1)	4 (7)	8 (4)	45 (75)	223 (95)
Compatible Philosophy and Objectives	5 (8)	18 (8)	6 (10)	39 (17)	49 (82)	171 (75)
Administrative Support	3 (5)	11 (5)	5 (8)	40 (17)	51 (87)	181 (78)
Effective Communication	3 (5)	6 (2)	8 (13)	18 (8)	49 (82)	209 (90)
Staff Number	0 (0)	4 (2)	5 (8)	19 (8)	55 (92)	209 (90)
Clinical Education Coordinator	0 (0)	2 (1)	5 (8)	19 (8)	55 (92)	211 (91)
Clinical Instructor Selection	5 (8)	14 (6)	6 (10)	25 (11)	49 (82)	194 (83)
Principles of Teaching and Learning	7 (12)	22 (9)	15 (25)	54 (23)	37 (63)	155 (68)
Sharing Special Expertise	1 (2)	4 (2)	12 (20)	15 (6)	47 (78)	214 (92)
Staff Development	10 (17)	7 (3)	17 (28)	37 (16)	33 (55)	186 (81)
Professional Associations	15 (25)	25 (11)	22 (37)	50 (22)	23 (38)	156 (67)
Internal Evaluation	19 (32)	18 (8)	22 (36)	52 (22)	19 (32)	163 (70)
Consumer Satisfaction	27 (45)	41 (18)	14 (24)	64 (27)	18 (31)	129 (55)
Personnel Roles	9 (15)	9 (4)	13 (21)	12 (5)	38 (64)	212 (91)
Support Services	7 (12)	28 (12)	12 (20)	37 (16)	40 (68)	165 (72)
Adequate Space	4 (7)	20 (9)	12 (20)	33 (14)	44 (73)	178 (77)

[a]Arranged in order of 1980 Standards.

[b]Rows do not sum to same number due to missing values.

C. 1. d Order

The identification of the crucial, as well as most and least important and practical, standards was also examined in the Weighting study. ACCEs and CCCEs participating in the study were asked if they believed any of the 1976 Standards were crucial (i.e., important or essential enough to cause dropping a center if not fulfilled). Ninety-four percent of the ACCEs and 91 percent of the CCCEs identified some of the 20 standards as crucial. The rank order of these standards is given in Table 5.

All participants in the study were asked to rank order the five most important and five least important standards, as well as the five most practical and five least practical standards. A non-parametric F test was used to test the significance of the differences, if any, in the rankings by the three samples: ACCEs, CCCEs (center), and CCCEs (academic). No significant differences in the rankings were found among the three samples at $p \leq .05$.

As can be seen in Table 5 the rank order of the standards for all three variables was similar in at least 10 standards (i.e., standards 1, 2, 6, 8, 9, 11, 12, 15, 16, and 19). A large spread between rankings occured in only a few cases (i.e., standards 5, 7, and 13).

Association between the variables, "importance" and "practicality," for each of the standards was checked by cross-tabulation tables. Chi-square tests showed that there is a significant association ($p \leq .05$) between the variables for each standard; while among the ACCEs, 13 standards (i.e., standards 3-8, 10, 11, 15, 16, 18-20) showed significant association.

Comparison of Tables 4 and 5 demonstrates that standards that were found more important, practical, and crucial were also found to be used more often by ACCEs and CCCEs.

TABLE 5

THE RANK ORDER OF THE CRUCIAL STANDARDS
AND THE COMPOSITE RANKING OF THE
STANDARDS ON IMPORTANCE AND PRACTICALITY[a]

Standard Key Words	Crucial	Importance	Practicality
1 Learning Environment	3	1	1
2 Program Planning	4	3	4
3 Learning Experiences	7	4	3
4 Ethical Standards	1	5	6
5 Affirmative Action	8	17	12
6 Compatible Philosophy and Objectives	5	6	8
7 Administrative Support	6	13	10
8 Effective Communication	9	8	9
9 Staff Number	2	2	2
10 Clinical Education Coordinator	10	7	5
11 Clinical Instructor Selection	11	11	14
12 Principles of Teaching and Learning	12	12	13
13 Sharing Special Expertise	19	9	7
14 Staff Development	16	10	11
15 Professional Associations	18	20	19
16 Internal Evaluation	15	14	16
17 Consumer Satisfaction	14	16	20
18 Personnel Roles	17	19	15
19 Support Services	20	18	18
20 Adequate Space	13	15	17

[a]Arranged in order of 1980 Standards.

C. 1. e Content Validity

     The Weighting study assessed the need to drop or add standards from or to the initial list of 20. Twenty-seven percent of the ACCEs and 22 percent of the CCCEs stated that some standards could be dropped. Standards 5--Affirmative Action, 15--Professional Associations, 16--Internal Evaluation, 17--Consumer Satisfaction, and 19--Support Services were specifically mentioned by 8 to 13 percent of the respondents. Eight percent of the ACCEs and five percent of the CCCEs suggested additional standards. Characteristics that were suggested already existed as part of one or more of the standards.

     In addition to these data from the Weighting study, data were collected in the Profile study concerning what ACCEs and CCCEs believe characterizes a "strong" clinical education center in physical therapy. Thirty-eight characteristics, or implicit standards, were listed. Eighteen of these characteristics were already directly included in the 20 1976 Standards. Content concerning "affirmative action" and "consumer satisfaction" mentioned in the Standards was not listed by ACCEs and CCCEs. Table 6 lists the remaining 20 characteristics that were not included verbatim in the 1976 Standards, but which could be matched with one of the Standards or its interpretation.

C. 1. f Discussion and Summary

     The 1976 Standards were examined in three studies: Pretest, Weighting, and Profile. Data from these studies were used to revise the Standards and interpretations. Except in the two cases mentioned below, the Standards were ordered according to the the data on crucial, important, and practical standards. "Staff Expertise" appeared as a part of the original standard concerning "Staff Number" (1980 Standard nine). Pretest data indicated that the original standard overlapped the content of another standard; therefore, data from the Weighting study were believed unreliable and were not used for this standard. The standard on "Affirmative Action" was placed in the top five because of the requirement that all federal facilities and facilities receiving federal funds abide by such a principle.

TABLE 6

CHARACTERISTICS OF A "STRONG" CLINICAL EDUCATION CENTER IN
PHYSICAL THERAPY NOT INCLUDED VERBATIM IN THE 1976 STANDARDS

Characteristic
Independent Practice
Evaluation of Students
Variety of Patients
Equipment
Balance in Variety of Learning Experiences
Orientation Program
Primary Patient Care
Treatment Techniques
Students from Several Schools
Convenient Geographical Location
Length of Affiliations
Written Agreements
PTs From Diversity of PT Schools
Methods
Physiatrist or MD Direction
Students to Improve and Challenge Staff
Community Acceptance
Accredited Institutions
PTA on Staff
Staff Accepted and Interested in PTA Program

Data showed that ACCEs and CCCEs believe that standards are needed to guide the selection and development of clinical education centers in physical therapy regardless of center size/type. Some of the standards are currently being used by ACCEs and CCCEs for these purposes.

This set of 20 Standards was the foundation for revision of the Self-Assessment and Student's forms and development of the Profile form. These evaluation forms were designed to measure compliance of a clinical education center with the Standards. The reliability and validity of these three forms are discussed in the next chapter.

II. D STUDIES OF EVALUATION FORMS

Measuring the variables that describe high quality clinical education is as difficult as any measurement in the behaviorial sciences.
Errors of measurement might play a larger role here than in the natu-
ral sciences, but attempts at evaluation are no less important. As
Kerlinger states when discussing evaluation in the behavioral sciences,
"We must always be very careful to ascertain the reliability and validity of our measures" (Kerlinger, 1979).

The clarity, practicality, usefulness, and content validity of
the 1976 Evaluation Forms were investigated in the Pretest. The content validity of the Self-Assessment form was also studied by the Project staff. The forms were revised based on the results of the Pretest and staff ratings. Reliability and validity of the revised evaluation forms were established based on results from the Interrater
Reliability and Internal Consistency studies. In the succeeding pages,
the order of the discussion will be as follows: results from the Pretest pertaining to clarity, practicality, usefulness, and content
validity of the 1976 Self-Assessment and Student's forms; data concerning the reliability of the revised forms; and data concerning
matched items on the revised Self-Assessment and Student's forms.

D. 1 Clarity, Practicality, Usefulness, and Content Validity of the
       1976 Evaluation Forms

       D. 1. a Self-Assessment Form

              Clarity, practicality, usefulness, and content
       validity of the 1976 Self-Assessment form were
       tested by the 28 CCCE participants in the Pretest.
       The participants unanimously stated that the instruc-
       tions for use of the Self-Assessment form were
       clearly written. Ten percent or more of the CCCEs
       stated that 55 (24%) of the 226 items on the Self-
       Assessment form needed to be revised for clarity,
       deleted, or placed elsewhere in the form. Sixty-one
       percent of the CCCE participants found the six hours
       required to complete the Self-Assessment form to be
       practical. Ninety-six percent of the CCCEs believed
       the Self-Assessment form would be useful in main-
       taining good communications with an educational pro-
       gram; 85 percent stated that the Self-Assessment
       would be useful in evaluating their clinical educa-
       tion program.

              The 1976 Self-Assessment form was also indepen-
       dently tested by three Project staff members and one
       Project consultant for content and construct vali-
       dity. Each item on the Self-Assessment form was

78

evaluated using specific guidelines. The judges
identified items that: 1) were not relevant to
clinical education, 2) did not measure a standard,
3) best measured each standard, and 4) might pre-
dict high quality clinical education. The responses of the judges were tabulated and discussed to
reach a consensus. The consensus items were included in the revised Self-Assessment form.

D. 1. b Student's Form

The clarity, practicality, usefulness, and
content validity of the 1976 Student's form was
tested in the Pretest. All 28 student participants
agreed that the instructions for use of the Student's form were clearly written. Eleven of the 34
items on the form were identified by at least 10
percent or more of the students as items to be
revised for clarity or deleted. The one hour
required to complete the Student's form was practical to 86 percent of the student participants. All
students, regardless of type of educational program
or length of affiliation, agreed that the Student's
form was useful in evaluating clinical education
centers and was appropriate for different sizes and
types of centers.

D. 2 Reliability of the 1980 Evaluation Forms

D. 2. a Self-Assessment Form

The interrater reliability of the Self-Assessment form was investigated in the Interrater Reliability study, the results of which are presented in
Table 7. In each of four centers, the CCCE and
several CIs independently filled out the Self-
Assessment form. Table 7 shows the proportion of
items on which all raters, or all but one of the
raters, agreed. These results are shown for each
of the centers and for all four centers combined.
The Self-Assessment form contains 213 items usable
in this approach to reliability. Thus, across the
four centers, there were 852 possible answers. On
646 of these possible answers, the raters were in
either total agreement or all but one of the raters
agreed. Thus, near perfect agreement was reached
75 percent of the time. On just over half of the
items (51%), the raters were in perfect agreement.

TABLE 7

INTERRATER RELIABILITY OF SELF-ASSESSMENT FORM

Standard Key Words[a]	Total # Items	Center A (n=4) T[b]	Center A n-1[c]	Center A %[d]	Center B (n=5) T	Center B n-1	Center B %	Center C (n=5) T	Center C n-1	Center C %	Center D (n=5) T	Center D n-1	Center D %	Across Centers (n=19) T	Across Centers n-1	Across Centers %
1 Learning Environment	16	8	4	75	6	0	37	7	6	81	4	3	43	25	13	59
2 Program Planning	25	16	6	88	17	5	88	18	4	88	19	5	96	70	20	90
3 Learning Experiences	4	2	2	100	3	3	100	4	0	100	1	1	100	10	6	100
4 Ethical Standards	11	11	0	100	8	3	100	7	4	100	5	1	54	31	8	89
5 Affirmative Action	5	4	1	100	4	1	100	4	0	80	4	0	80	16	2	90
6 Compatible Philosophy and Objectives	12	10	0	83	10	1	83	9	3	100	6	2	66	35	6	85
7 Administrative Support	12	5	5	83	7	2	75	9	2	92	4	4	66	25	13	79
8 Effective Communication	2	0	2	100	2	0	100	0	2	100	0	2	100	4	6	100
9 Staff Number	5	0	2	40	4	0	80	0	1	20	0	4	80	4	7	55
10 Clinical Education Coordinator	1	1	0	100	1	0	100	1	0	100	1	0	100	4	0	100
11 Clinical Instructor Selection	1	1	0	100	1	0	100	1	0	100	1	0	100	4	0	100
12 Principles of Teaching and Learning	11	3	6	82	4	2	54	5	4	82	2	8	91	14	20	77
13 Sharing Special Expertise	7	3	2	71	1	3	57	2	1	43	0	3	43	6	9	54
14 Staff Development	8	2	6	100	4	1	62	8	0	100	3	4	87	17	11	87
15 Professional Associations	13	2	0	15	0	2	15	1	1	7	3	0	23	6	3	17
16 Internal Evaluation	24	14	8	92	14	6	25	13	1	54	7	7	29	48	22	73
17 Consumer Satisfaction	13	10	3	100	9	2	100	3	6	69	8	5	100	30	18	92
18 Personnel Roles	6	6	0	100	3	4	83	6	0	100	2	3	83	17	5	61
19 Support Services	28	16	6	78	14	6	71	17	5	76	12	9	75	59	26	76
20 Adequate Space	9	1	5	66	5	4	100	4	4	44	2	3	55	12	16	77
TOTAL	213	115	58	81	115	45	77	119	44	77	86	64	70	435	211	76

[a] Arranged in order of 1980 Standards.
[b] T indicated total (perfect) agreement among respondents.
[c] n-1 indicated all but one respondent agreed (near perfect agreement) on item.
[d] Percent represents the proportion of the items per standard with perfect or near perfect agreement among respondents (e.g., using the data for Center A, for the standard concerning the Learning Environment, 12 divided by 16 equals .75 or 75%).

Some standards were found to be more reliable among raters than others. Perfect or near perfect agreement was reached only 17 percent of the time for standard 15--Professional Associations; while several standards showed perfect or near-perfect agreement 100 percent of the time (3, 8, 10, and 11) and three others were at or above ninety percent (2, 5, and 17). Of the 20 Standards, 14 showed complete or near-perfect agreement, at least 75% of the time. Thus, within centers, there appears to be a very high level of agreement on the revised Self-Assessment form.

Table 8 presents the results of the internal consistency calculations using the RELIABILITY subprogram of Statistical Package for the Social Science (SPSS). This subprogram allows one to compute Cronbach's Alpha and shows the effect on Alpha of deleting each item from the standard. For example, if a particular item correlates negatively with the total score, Alpha will increase when that item is removed from the standard. The results shown in Table 8 are based on standards from which those items that did not vary, and in a few cases those that have low correlations with total score, have been removed. The results are based on fifty observations.

Using the generally accepted rule of .6 as an adequate level of reliability, 12 of the 16 standards for which Alpha can be estimated are acceptable. Two standards did not show sufficient variance to allow an estimation of reliability and two standards contained only one item. Four of the standards showed unacceptably low Alphas. Two of them, standard 13--Sharing Special Expertise and standard 15--Professional Associations, also have low percent of interrater agreement. Thus, some attempt to write additional items to measure these concepts or to clarify existing items may be appropriate.

TABLE 8

INTERNAL CONSISTENCY OF SELF-ASSESSMENT FORM

Standard Key Words[a]	Total Number of Items Per Standard	Number of Items Per Standard with Zero Variance[b]	Alpha[c]
Learning Environment	15	2	.71041
Program Planning	24	2	.75763
Learning Experiences	5	5	...[d]
Ethical Standards	11	0	.75645
Affirmative Action	5	4	...
Compatible Philosophy and Objectives	11	0	.65274
Administrative Support	7	0	.64682
Effective Communication	102	1	.90781
Staff Number	5	0	.54507
Clinical Education Coordinator	1	1	...
Clinical Instructor Selection	1	1	...
Principles of Teaching and Learning	12	0	.70671
Sharing Special Expertise	8	1	.37152
Staff Development	7	0	.63411
Professional Associations	5	0	.42716
Internal Evaluation	23	1	.66081
Consumer Satisfaction	14	0	.66579
Personnel Roles	6	0	.53880
Support Services	27	0	.62397
Adequate Space	9	0	.69940

D. 2. b Profile Form

The interrater reliability of the revised Profile form was studied in the Interrater Reliability study conducted in four centers. One CCCE and four CIs in each center were asked to complete this form. The twenty items on the graphic portion of the Profile form were checked for their reliability. Analysis of the form included assessing reliability of the form across centers and then within centers. Results presented in Table 9 demonstrate that the Profile form is reliable across raters and centers.

In the analysis across centers, the form was found to be reliable with an Alpha of .89177. Likewise, analysis of the form within centers demonstrated that it was reliable even though the reliability within each center is somewhat lower than the composite for the four centers. This finding can be explained by the small number of respondents from each center.

---

[a] Arranged in order of 1980 Standards.
[b] The RELIABILITY subprogram from Statistical Package for the Social Sciences (SPSS) was used to analyze the reliability of the Self-Assessment, the Profile, and the Student's forms. Reliability is defined as the ratio of true score variance to total variance over an indefinitely large number of independent, repeated trials (Nie, Hull, Jenkins, et al, 1977). Items with no variance (i.e., items on which the respondents completely agree) are reliable by definition. The subprogram computes the reliability of scales based only on those items that have variance.
[c] The reliability coefficient denoted by Alpha, can vary from zero to one depending on the amount of measurement error. A value of .6 or above is typically accepted as indicative of reasonable reliability (Robinson, Athanasion, Head, 1969).
[d] Ellipses indicate little or no variance in responses.

Note: The above explanations also pertain to Tables 9 and 10.

TABLE 9

RELIABILITY OF THE PROFILE FORM[a]

	Total Number of Items	Total Number of Items with Zero Variance	Alpha
All 4 centers (19 respondents)	20	0	.89177
Center A (3 respondents)	20	2	.68897
Center B (5 respondents)	20	11	.70734
Center C (5 respondents)	20	0	.60415
Center D (4 respondents)	20	2	.80878

[a] *See Table 8 for explanation of zero variance and Alpha.*

As shown in Table 9 two items out of 20 did not have variance in Center A, 11 items did not have variance in Center B, and two items did not have variance in Center D. Therefore, these items were not included in the calculation of the reliability for each of these centers. They are reliable by definition.

D. 2. c Student's Form

The Student's form was studied in the Interrater Reliability study. In each of the centers, five students who were assigned to the center at the time of the study were asked to complete a revised Student's form. The results of this study were analyzed in three stages: first, the reliability of the whole form across centers was examined, then the reliability of the form was studied according to topics of common interest within the form (e.g., Orientation) both across and within centers. Table 10 presents the results of the reliability study across and within centers according to topics of common interest on the form.

84

The revised Student's form was found reliable. The analysis of the whole form across centers included 98 items. Nineteen out of the 98 items had zero variance; the other 79 items showed a reliability coefficient of .84757.

As can be seen in Table 10, two topics--Supervision and Evaluation--were found to be most reliable. Nine items out of 10 in the Supervision category and three items out of four in the Evaluation category have zero variance in all four centers (i.e., all participants gave the same responses to these items).

The other topics were found reliable in analysis across centers. The small n per center explains the variability in α. For example, on the topic, Orientation, α varies among the 4 centers from -.13 to .91. Therefore, responses were aggregated across centers to estimate what α would be with a larger n per center. This aggregated α reflects between center variance, but is an acceptable estimate of α with a large n.

TABLE 10

RELIABILITY OF THE STUDENT'S FORM ACCORDING TO TOPICS OF COMMON INTEREST[a]

Topics of Common Interest in the Student's Form	All 4 Centers (19 Respondents)			Center A (5 Respondents)		Center B (5 Respondents)		Center C (4 Respondents)		Center D (5 Respondents)	
	Total Number of Items for Each Topic	Total Number of Items With Zero Variance	Alpha	Total Number of Items With Zero Variance	Alpha	Total Number of Items With Zero Variance	Alpha	Total Number of Items With Zero Variance	Alpha	Total Number of Items With Zero Variance	Alpha
Information	29	1	.83219	7	.72738	11	.91996	8	.94610	11	.64087
Orientation	13	0	.71980	3	.84362	5	-.12698	6	.45370	4	.90900
Learning	40	6	.78369	14	.86434	25	.61071	21	.89106	18	.79896
Supervision	10	9	...	10	...	9	...	10	...	10	...
Evaluation	4	3	...	3	...	3	...	3	...	4	...

[a] See Table 8 for explanation of zero variance, Alpha, and ellipses.

86

D. 3 Matches Between Student and Clinical Staff Responses

Twenty-five items on the Student's form closely or exactly matched items on the Self-Assessment form. By comparing the responses from the two groups to these items, insight into the reliability and validity of the forms can be gained. If the responses are in perfect agreement, it can be argued that the forms are both reliable and valid in that respondents appear to come to the same evaluation (reliability) and we can assume that the shared evaluation is based on the same interpretation of the item (validity). On the other hand, if there is not agreement between students and clinical staff, it may reflect random error (unreliability) on the part of one or both groups or disagreement between the two groups as to the meaning of the items (invalidity).

The results show that on about two-thirds (68%) of the items there is at least 75 percent agreement between the two groups of raters. For 40 percent of the 25 similar items, there was complete agreement between students and clinical staff. For about a third of the items, there was less than 75 percent agreement. Since the results of the earlier studies suggest that the items are reasonably reliable on both the Student's and the Self-Assessment forms, the low degree of agreement on some of the items would suggest that students are unfamiliar with some of the concepts relating to administrative precedures, personnel policies, and other similar matters.

D. 4 Discussion and Summary

Reliability of the 1980 forms to evaluate clinical education centers was studied in the Interrater Reliability and Internal Consistency studies. These two studies differed in three major points. While in the Interrater Reliability study the reliability of the three forms within centers was examined by asking respondents with similar backgrounds to evaluate their center with the same evaluation forms, the Internal Consistency study examined only the reliability of the Self-Assessment form across centers. A second major difference between the studies was that for the Interrater Reliability study the Self-Assessment form was independently completed by one CCCE and four CIs, who because of their different positions could be assumed to have different perceptions of the center; in the Internal Consistency study, only the CCCE in each center completed a Self-Assessment form. A third difference between the studies was that the random sample drawn for the Internal Consistency study offered the potential for including all sizes and types of centers, while only large centers were selected for the Interrater Reliability study.

II. E   RELIABILITY AND VALIDITY OF EVALUATION PROCESS

The evaluation process based on the use of the revised Standards, Self-Assessment and Profile forms was examined for reliability and validity in the Test phase which included 17 centers. Reliability was investigated by comparing repeated measures of the same variable across raters (staff and ACCE); and validity, by comparing relationships between two different measures of clinical center quality. Results of the Test phase were expressed as scores which were derived for each center by averaging all ACCE or Staff ratings of that center. Six sets of scores for the 17 centers were correlated. These six scores (Table 11) represent: the raters (staff or ACCE); the variables measured (Compliance with the standards obtained by averaging the ratings on a completed Profile form, or overall Strength of the clinical education program measured on a scale of 1 to 20); and the conditions under which the ratings were made (with Self-Assessment information and no identity of the center or CCCE, or with identity of the CCCE and center and no Self-Assessment information available). The correlation matrix is shown in Table 12. Each cell of the matrix is referred to by a lower case Arabic letter. All but four of the fifteen correlations are statistically significant, $p \leq .003$. (p=.05 divided by 15 nonindependent variables.)

E. 1   Parallel-Test Model

Correlations a, b, c, j, n, and o demonstrate reliability in the sense that they are parallel measures of the same variable (Nunnally, 1978), either Compliance (r_a, r_b, r_c) or Strength (r_j, r_n, r_o). These correlations show that the greatest consistency in ratings occured when different raters used the Self-Assessment information to rate the centers (r_a, r_j). Inconsistencies in ratings were greater when the raters and the conditions varied (r_b, r_n), and when the ACCEs rated under two different conditions (r_c, r_o).

TABLE 11

DESCRIPTION OF EACH SCORE USED IN THE TEST

Scores	Variables		Raters		Conditions	
	Compliance[a]	Strength[b]	Staff	ACCE	With Self-Assessment Information; No CCCE Identity (Condition I)	No Self-Assessment Information; With CCCE Identity (Condition II)
Staff Compliance Score	X		X		X	
ACCE Compliance Score I	X			X	X	
ACCE Compliance Score II	X			X		X
Staff Strength Score		X	X		X	
ACCE Strength Score I		X		X	X	
ACCE Strength Score II		X		X		X

[a] Compliance with the standards.
[b] Overall strength of the clinical education center.

TABLE 12

CORRELATION MATRIX OF TEST RESULTS

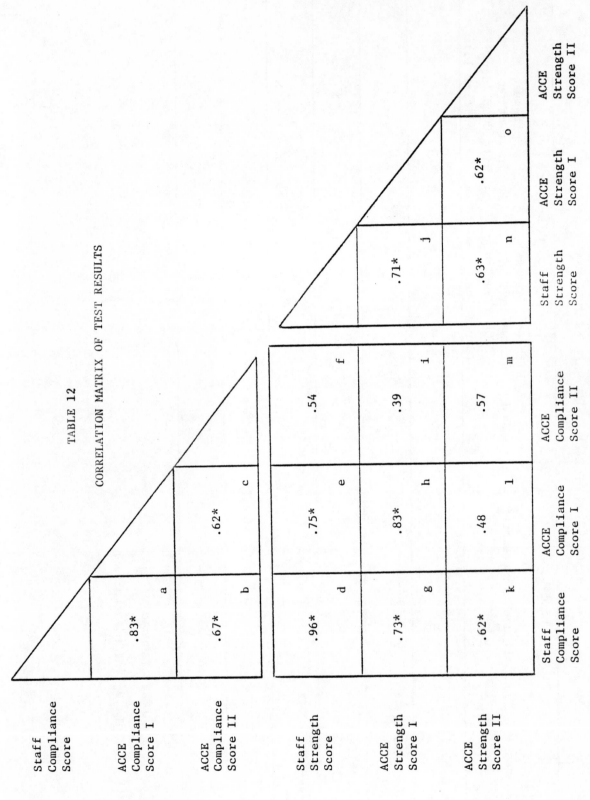

	Staff Compliance Score	ACCE Compliance Score I	ACCE Compliance Score II	Staff Strength Score	ACCE Strength Score I
ACCE Compliance Score I	.83* (a)				
ACCE Compliance Score II	.67* (b)	.62* (c)			
Staff Strength Score	.96* (d)	.75* (e)	.54 (f)		
ACCE Strength Score I	.73* (g)	.83* (h)	.39 (i)	.71* (j)	
ACCE Strength Score II	.62* (k)	.48 (l)	.57 (m)	.63* (n)	.62* (o)

*significant at $p < .003$; $p=.05$ divided by 15 nonindependent variables. The small letter in the bottom right corner of each cell is used to identify the cell.

The remaining nine correlations in the matrix (i.e., correlations d, e, f, g, h, i, k, 1, and m) demonstrate validity in the sense that they show relationships between the two different measurement variables, Compliance and Strength, across various measurement conditions and raters. The pattern obvious throughout these nine correlations was similar to that shown by the reliability estimates. The correlations were highest when Self-Assessment information was used to guide the ratings (Table 13). This held true whether the raters varied or were constant, or whether the measures varied or were held constant.

TABLE 13

CORRELATIONS BY CONDITIONS AND RATERS

Same Conditions				Different Conditions	
Self-Assessment Information (Condition I)		No Self-Assessment Information (Condition II)			
Same Raters	Different Raters	Same Raters	Different Raters	Same Raters	Different Raters
r_d .96	r_a .83	r_m .57		r_c .62	r_b .67
r_h .83	r_e .75			r_o .62	r_n .63
	r_g .73			r_1 .48	r_k .62
	r_j .71			r_i .39	r_f .54

Means and variances of the six variables were examined to determine the effect of using the Self-Assessment information to rate a center (Table 14). The magnitude of the difference in means and variances was not statistically significant for either the Compliance scores or the Strength scores ($p > .05$). However, the scores obtained under Condition II, with no Self-Assessment information available (ACCE Compliance Score II, ACCE Strength Score II) tended to show slightly higher means and lower variances than those scores performed with Self-Assessment information available (Staff Compliance Score, Staff Strength Score, ACCE Compliance Score I, ACCE Strength Score I). The lower means and higher variances obtained when the Self-Assessment information was used indicates that this condition allows a less biased and more discriminating evaluation of a center.

TABLE 14

MEANS AND VARIANCES OF SCORES BY CONDITIONS

Score/Condition	Compliance[a]		Score/Condition	Strength[b]	
	Mean	Variance		Mean	Variance
Condition I Scores:			Condition I Scores:		
Staff Compliance	7.45	.445	Staff Strength	13.588	7.854
ACCE Compliance	7.62	.578	ACCE Strength	15.230	8.477
Condition II Scores:			Condition II Scores:		
ACCE Compliance	7.97	.479	ACCE Strength	16.509	4.255

[a]Compliance score obtained by averaging ratings on completed Profile form.
[b]Strength score obtained by rating a center on a scale of 1 to 20.

92

The analysis of the data as presented thus far follows the classical definitions of reliability and validity as described by the parallel-test model. This is a more stringent test of the reliability of the revised Self-Assessment and Profile forms than reported earlier in the Interrater Reliability and Internal Consistency tests of the forms because additional sources of variance have been introduced.

E. 2 True-Score Model

Data from the Test phase were further analyzed in accordance with the true-score model of test theory. This approach is based on the assumption that an error free score (i.e., true score) exists and can be ascertained. Such a score can then serve as a valid criterion to which other scores can be compared.

In the Test phase, the Staff Scores on Compliance and Strength can be assumed to be true scores. This assumption is tenable because staff members have worked together to revise the standards and evaluation forms and share interpretations of each of the standards. Further support is evident in the high staff interrater reliability coefficients (.71 to .89) and the extremely high correlation (r_d .96) between Staff Scores on compliance and strength reported earlier.

Analysis of the Test data, from the perspective of the true-score model, show that ACCEs' scores correlate with the true score more highly when they have information from a completed Self-Assessment form to guide their ratings (See correlations a and b; j and n in Table 12). (A more complete discussion of the logic of this analysis can be found in the final report of the Project.)

E. 3 Discussion and Summary

The results of this study clearly demonstrate the reliability of the clinical education center evaluation process using the 1980 Standards, Self-Assessment and Profile forms. The correlations between parallel measures of the same variable were higher when the raters had Self-Assessment information to guide their ratings, than when they did not. These data suggest that use of the Self-Assessment and the Profile forms can lead to a reliable evaluation of a clinical education center. Validity of the evaluation process was demonstrated by the high correlation between the Compliance and Strength scores when these scores were based on Self-Assessment information. Judgments based on such information are closer to a true, error free evaluation than are judgments made without the Self-Assessment information.

II. F INQUIRES

Requests concerning raw data or questionnaires or any other information about the Project should be directed to:

Institute for Research in Social Science
Manning Hall
University of North Carolina at Chapel Hill
Chapel Hill, North Carolina 27514

REFERENCES

Barr, JS, Gwyer, J, Talmor Z: A method for developing clinical education standards with evaluation forms: A project in progress, 1980a. (Submitted to Evaluation and the Health Professions)

Barr JS, Gwyer J, Talmor Z: Evaluation of clinical education in physical therapy, 1980b. (Submitted to Physical Therapy)

Barr JS, Gwyer J, Talmor Z: Project on Selection of Clinical Education Sites. Final Report. Washington, Department of Health, Education, and Welfare, Allied Health Special Project, 1980c

Kerlinger F: Behavioral Research: A Conceptual Approach. New York, Holt, Rinehart and Winston, 1979, p 62

Moore ML, Perry JF: Clinical Education in Physical Therapy: Present Status/ Future Needs. Washington, American Physical Therapy Association, 1976

Nie NH, Hull CH, Jenkins JG, et al: Statistical Package for the Social Sciences. New York, McGraw Hill Book Company, Update manual, March, 1977

Nunnally JC: Psychometric Theory, ed 2: New York, McGraw-Hill Book Company, 1978

Robinson JP, Athanasiou R, Head K: Measures of occupational attitudes and occupational characteristics. Ann Arbor, The University of Michigan, Institute for Social Research, 1969

SUGGESTED READINGS

Moore ML, Perry JF: Clinical Education in The Health Professions: An Annotated Bibliography. Washington, American Physical Therapy Association, 1976

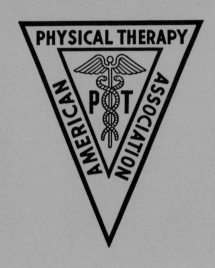